THERAPEUTIC FASTING

THERAPEUTIC

FASTING

BY

ARNOLD DE VRIES

TABLE OF CONTENTS

THERAPEUTIC FASTING

⋏ I ⋏

Forms of Fasting

THE TERM, fasting, implies total or partial abstinence from food or water for any of a number of reasons. Thus one may refer to fruit fasts, vegetable fasts, milk fasts, water fasts and many other types. As the different reasons for fasting are considered, other divisions may be given—viz, religious fasting, professional fasting, physiological fasting, pathological fasting and accidental or experimental fasting.

A fruit fast is abstinence from fruit; a vegetable fast is abstinence from vegetables; a milk fast is abstinence from milk; a water fast is abstinence from water, and similar fasts may be defined accordingly. Religious fasting is abstinence to develop spiritual thought or fulfill a religious rite. Professional fasting is abstinence for purposes of notoriety and publicity. Physiological fasting is normal inanition in nature, such as the hibernation and seasonal abstinence of certain animals. Pathological fasting is associated with organic derangements which make one unable to take or retain food. Accidental or experimental fasting is forced inanition among man or animals for purposes of scientific investigation.

These are the recognized forms of fasting. Yet, there is another, and perhaps much more important, classification which is seldom given mention or even known about. This is therapeutic fasting—total abstinence from all food, but not water. The purpose of therapeutic fasting is the promotion and restoration of health. It is associated with experimental and physiological fasting in the sense that studies of the latter provide the knowledge and information which make therapeutic fasting possible.

Therapeutic fasting is not the result of any particular new scientific discovery, but rather has proceeded to its present development as the result of centuries of experimentation, observation and study. It is today the culmination of a large number of scientific investigations and discoveries which have reached their climax during the past century. Fasting for therapeutic purposes is thus an important, though in popular conception, almost unknown, phase of the modern science of medicine, and as such it is the subject of our present inquiry and analysis.

❧ II ❧

A Short History of Fasting

THE ORIGIN OF FASTING for illness perhaps dates back to the development of the present forms of animal life. Among undomesticated animals it is a common practice to fast when ill, though this is of course an instinctive procedure rather than a planned therapeutic measure. The first records of human fasting for the remedy of disease go back to the ancient civilizations of Greece and the Near East. Both Plato and Socrates are said to have fasted for 10 days at a time to "attain mental and physical efficiency." Pythagoras fasted for 40 days before taking his examination at the University of Alexandria, and then he also required his pupils to fast before they could enter his class. The ancient Egyptians were said to treat syphilis with their fasting cures, and the great Greek physician, Hippocrates, prescribed fasting during the critical periods of disease. Asclepiades and Thessalus employed fasting; Celsus is said to have used it in the treatment of jaundice and epilepsy, and the Arab physician, Avicenna, prescribed fasting for three to five weeks at a time. Later Tertullian wrote of fasting, and Plutarch said: "Instead of using medicine better fast a day."

During the sixteenth century, the renowned Swiss physician, Paracelsus, claimed that, "Fasting is the greatest remedy." In the seventeenth century, Dr. Hoffman wrote a book entitled, *Description of the Magnificent Results Obtained Through Fasting in All Diseases*. Dr. Anton Nikolai followed in the next century with recommendations of fasting instead of food for those who were ill. Later Dr. Von Seeland, of Russia, wrote: "As a result of experiments I have come to the conclusion that fasting is not only a therapeutic of the highest degree possible but also deserves consideration educationally." In Germany, Dr. Adolph Mayer asserted that "fasting is the most efficient means of correcting any disease," and Dr. Moeller wrote that "fasting is the only natural evolutionary method whereby through a systemic cleansing you can restore yourself by degrees to physiologic normality."

It has been during the past century that the greater portion of scientific data has been gathered. Both Europe (in particular, Germany) and America have contributed heavily to the research on experimental and physiological fasting. Hundreds of publications have been the result of this work and they provide thorough and exact knowledge regarding many phases of fasting. Among the best known research scientists who studied fasting were: Sergius Morgulis, Professor of Biochemistry at the University of Nebraska College of Medicine; Professor Child, of the University of Chicago; Herbert Sidney Langfield, of Harvard University; Dr. Frederick M. Allen, of the Rockefeller Institute; Francis Gano Benedict and Ernest G. Ritzman, of the Carnegie Institute; Luigi Luciani, Professor of Physiology at the University of Rome; and Victor Pashutin, Director of the Imperial Military Medical Academy of pre-revolutionary Russia. Other scientific studies of fasting have been made by N. Pyaskovski, W. Skorczewski, N. J. Sands, A. Cleghorn, N. Morozov, P. B. Hawk, P. E. Howe, O. S. Soltz, C. A. Stewart, S. R. Wreath, C. M. Jackson, L. H. Hyman, N. Zuntz, Roger et Josue, Miescher, Mansfield, Rosenfeld and many others. All told, during the past century, hundreds of scientific workers in many countries have added to our knowledge of the biological importance of fasting.

In contrast to these scientists, who were concerned primarily with developing laboratory data from studies of experimental and physiological fasting, chiefly among animals and to a lesser extent among humans, we have the other men of science who were concerned with the clinical and therapeutic phases of fasting. They supervised tens of thousands of fasts, and as a result discovered the exact effectiveness of fasting as a remedy for specific diseases. Among these physicians were many of the nineteenth century, in addition to those now practicing. They include, among others: Dr. Isaac Jennings, Dr. Joel Shew, Dr. Russell Thacker Trall, Dr. Robert Walter, Dr. Henry S. Tanner, and Dr. Edward Hooker Dewey. The experience of these men was followed in the twentieth century by that of Dr. Linda Burfield Hazzard; Dr. Hereward Carrington; Dr. Eugene A. Bergholtz, of Milwaukee, Wisconsin; Dr. John M. Tilden, of Denver, Colorado; Dr. William Howard Hay, of Mount Pocana, Pennsylvania, and Dr. George S. Weger, of Redlands, California. Today Dr. Herbert M. Shelton, of San Antonio, Texas, carries on the important work, and Doctors Esser, Benesh, McEachen, Gross, and Scott are also making important contributions.

History thus affords evidence of the considerable amount of scientific and clinical work done to determine the effects of fasting. The therapeutic measure is not a new and untried method, but on the contrary has been recognized for centuries and has been studied by some of the most brilliant minds in the science of medicine and related fields. The importance of these studies may be readily seen upon examination of the unique record of fasting, as regards its curative influence in the case of many specific diseases. A careful scientific appraisal of therapeutic fasting may then be of significance to both the physician and layman.

❧ III ❧

Physiological Reactions to Fasting

THE DEVELOPMENT AND EVOLUTION of the forms of human pathology are governed by the physiological and chemical reactions that are taking place. Anything that induces such reactions plays a role in determining the state of human health. Whenever food is withheld from consumption beyond the usual period in the case of man or other animals there are certain changes in the function, chemical reactions and life processes of the cells and tissues. It is these changes which give fasting its therapeutic properties. By considering the physiological reactions to fasting we can thus gain an understanding of the reasons which determine its therapeutic value.

Of great importance among the physiological effects of fasting is rejuvenescence—the acquiring of fresh vitality and renewal of youthful characteristics to the cells and tissues of the body. Evidence of such regeneration comes from many quarters and is particularly impressing with respect to experimental work done with the various forms of lower animal life. Such work may then be given first consideration.

The British scientist, Prof. Huxley, has carried out experiments with young planaria, more commonly known as earthworms. He fed an entire colony of these worms their usual foods. One of the worms was isolated from the rest and fasted at periodic intervals. In all other respects its diet and mode of life were similar to those of the other worms. The isolated worm lived while 19 generations of worms in the colony lived and passed away.

Prof. Child, of the University of Chicago, likewise has used worms to determine the effects of fasting. He took a group of small flat worms which had grown old and infirm and fasted them for months, until they had been reduced to a minimum size. Then he started feeding them again, and as they grew back to their normal size, they were just as young, from a physiological standpoint, as they ever were. In his *Senescence and Rejuvenescence*, Prof. Child remarks: "Partial starvation inhibits senescence. The starveling is brought back from an advanced age to the beginning of post-embryonic life; it is almost reborn."

Other experiments, conducted by E. Schultz, have shown that hydra are rejuvenated by fasting, the animals reverting back to an embryonic state. At the University of Chicago, one insect, the normal life span of which is one day, was fasted and lived for 15 days. There are some species of lower animal life which normally pass through their life span in three or four weeks, but when, because of lack of food, they are forced to fast at intervals, they often remain young and active for three years.

Prof. Sergius Morgulis, in his experimental work with animals, has noted the relation between fasting and rejuvenation. He states: "Laboratory as well as clinical experiments corroborated the rejuvenating effects of inanition. If it is not too prolonged it is distinctly beneficent and may well be used in over-coming somnolence and lassitude as well as in improving the fundamental organic functions (circulation, respiration), muscular strength, or the acuity of the senses. . . . Biologically speaking, though the organism acquires no new assets it becomes stronger by ridding itself of liabilities. In the foregoing it has been pointed out that the cell-nucleus ratio changes in such a manner as to increase the preponderance of the nucleus. Morphologically, therefore, the cells composing the entire organism assume a more youthful condition. They resemble more the embryonic cells in this respect, and this may account for the expansive growth which they display under the proper nutritive regime."

One of the characteristics of old age is a decrease in the metabolic rate. It is interesting to note, in this connection, that fasting produces rejuvenation by inducing a permanent increase in the metabolic rate. In experiments conducted at the Hull Biological Laboratory of the University of Chicago, both dogs and humans were fasted for extended periods. In fasts of from 30 to 40 days a five to six per cent increase in the metabolic rate was observed.

Of course rejuvenation does not occur in man to the extent that it does in the lowest forms of animal life. However, the effects of rejuvenescence are nevertheless very noticeable in the case of human fasting. Dr. Carlson and Dr. Kunde, of the Department of Physiology in the University of Chicago, placed a 40 year old man on a 14 days fast. At the end of the fast his tissues were in the same physiological condition as those of a 17 year old youth. In reference to fasting Dr. Kunde remarks: "It is evident that where the initial weight was reduced by 45 per cent, and subsequently restored by normal diet, approximately one-half of the restored body is made up of new protoplasm. In this there is rejuvenescence." It may also be pointed out that quite possibly much of the remaining part of the body not lost in weight may also undergo significant changes of rejuvenescence as a result of fasting.

Mention may also be given to the case of the late Mahatma Gandhi, who was well known for his numerous fasts. On May 18, 1933, when Gandhi was in the tenth day of fasting, he was examined by his physicians. One of the physicians stated that "despite his 64 years, from a physiological point of view the Indian leader was as healthy as a man of forty."

The outward manifestations of regeneration are quite noticeable in many cases of fasting. The rejuvenating effect upon the skin in particular is important. Lines and wrinkles become less apparent, and blotches, discolorations and pimples tend to disappear. In the words of Dr. Shelton: "The skin becomes more youthful, acquires a better color and better texture. The eyes clear up and become brighter. One looks younger. The visible rejuvenation in the skin is matched by manifest evidences of similar but invisible rejuvenescence throughout the body."

Literally the word, autolysis, means self-loosing. In physiology it is used to denote the process of digestion or disintegration of animal tissue by ferments and enzymes which are generated by the body cells themselves. Thus it is a process of self-digestion or intra-cellular digestion.

Autolysis forms a normal part of the physiological activities of the body. The action of enzymes upon such substances in the body as glycogen, fatty tissue and bone marrow, in preparing these materials for entry into the blood stream, is normal autolysis. Likewise when an abscess "points" to the surface of the body to empty its contents, autolysis was involved when the flesh between the abscess and the surface was digested by enzymes.

While recognizing the existence of autolysis as a common fact of everyday life, it has been generally believed that the process could not be made subject to human control and put to practical use. Though it has been understood that abnormal growths in the body might be absorbed through self-disintegration, the profound change in metabolism necessary to bring about such autolysis has been thought to result only in very rare cases following such conditions as extreme cachexia, the puerperium, or menopause. Such conditions, not always being within the realm of voluntary control, and only occasionally producing the changes in question, offer no method whereby autolysis can be instituted at will and put under control.

A complete revolution in such orthodox concepts necessarily follows consideration of fasting. The fact is that fasting, in producing a profound change in metabolism, serves as an immediate inducement to the development of autolysis and can thus act as a control of this process. This is no new discovery in physiology, but has been recognized for over a century by those who employed fasting. In the early part of the nineteenth century, Sylvester Graham wrote that "it is a general law of the vital economy" that "the decomposing absorbents always first lay hold of and remove those substances which are of least use to the economy; and hence, all morbid accumulations, such as wens, tumors, abscesses, etc., are rapidly diminished and often wholly removed under severe and protracted abstinence and fasting."

During the fast, the body has the opportunity to redistribute its nutritive supplies—the surpluses and non-vital supplies being consumed and utilized first. The absorption of normal muscles and tissues on a fast is readily observable, and the flesh, blood and bone of a tumor, being less important to the needs of the body, are absorbed much more rapidly, with the essential tissues being utilized in nourishment and the remainder permanently removed.

On the fast the assimilative powers of the body are increased. This is shown both in the improvement of the blood during the fast and the rapid assimilation of food after the fast. Patients who suffer from conditions such as anemia, with either an insufficiency of red blood cells or an excess of white cells, are generally normalized by fasting. In some cases fasting has brought about an increase in the number of erythrocytes from only one million to the normal five million count. The explanation lies in the improvement in assimilation which the fast affords. The iron and other elements which are stored in the body are taken up by the blood and used. Prior to fasting, general physiological inefficiency prevented this. Perhaps this also explains why dental decay is often arrested during the fast. In some cases teeth that were loose become firmly fixed in their sockets while fasting, and swollen, inflamed and bleeding gums are also restored to health. The improvement in assimilation during the fast actually brings about recovery of certain "deficiency" diseases.

Assimilation after the fast is at the highest possible level. Kagan observed that after rabbits were fasted 17 days they gained 56 per cent in weight on a diet which, under usual conditions, would barely be sufficient to maintain a state of equilibrium. People who are chronically underweight in spite of eating very heavily, often gain weight to the normal level after a fast, even though large quantities of food are not taken. The improved assimilation enables the body to utilize more of its food intake.

It may be mentioned that it is really a *normalization* of assimilation which occurs on a fast. Patients who fast to rid themselves of excessive weight may gain weight to normal after the fast, but that is usually where the gain ends if nutrition is proper. Thus both people who assimilate too much of their food intake, and those who assimilate too little, are helped by fasting.

Fasting affords the organs of the body the closest possible approach to a complete physiological rest. Many organs are overworked and overstimulated, and hence weakened, through the constant use of defective foods and excessive quantities of foods. During a fast, the necessary work done by the organs is reduced to the lowest possible minimum. As there is no further intake of food, assimilation in the body only involves the redistribution of the elements already stored there. Thus the organs are given a chance to recuperate and restore their vital powers. Repair of damaged structures may take place. Broken bones, wounds and open sores heal much more rapidly. If inflammation is present it tends to subside. The body undergoes a general healing process.

Associated with physiological rest of an organ is increased elimination. This, according to some observers, is the most important advantage of fasting. Part of the energy which would normally be devoted to the work of assimilation may, during a fast, be used to expel the accumulations of waste and toxins. Decomposing food in the digestive tract, which is often an important source of toxins, is quickly eliminated.

The entire alimentary canal becomes almost free from bacteria. The nourishment of cells on a fast is first derived from the less essential tissues and portions of impaired and diseased tissue. The surplus material on hand is utilized first. The effusions, dropsical swellings, fat, infiltrations, etc., are absorbed with great rapidity on a fast. The body thus gradually releases itself from a former burden of superfluous and waste material.

Increased elimination of toxins is noted on the very first days of the fast. The breath becomes very offensive, and the skin may also emit an offensive odor, possibly because of greater eliminative effort on the part of both the lungs and skin. Catarrhal eliminations usually increase during the early days of the fast, until towards the end of the fast elimination is completed and recovery occurs. The toxicity of the urine is increased, perhaps due to greater elimination via the kidneys. In some cases, considerable waste material is lost through the process of vomiting. Of course each of these symptoms does not occur in all cases, but there is always some outward indication of increased elimination. The primary elimination, however, brought about simply by internal absorption and autolysis, is not apparent in outward reactions, except perhaps the loss of weight and general weakness.

A marked improvement in nervous and mental function occurs on the fast. Max Nordau declared that "Pessimism has a physiological basis," and it may also be said that even the most severe forms of mental aberration usually have a physiological basis. Under the usual circumstances of civilized life, with its nutritive inadequacies and its inclusion of chemical stimulants and depressants, both in the food supply and as drugs for the treatment of disease, there is a tendency to the reduction of nerve energy, or enervation as it is called. The capacity of the brain is also impaired, giving rise to an assortment of nervous and mental diseases. While fasting, all enervating influences are discontinued and the entire nervous system and brain undergoes the same physiological rest that the balance of the body experiences. Nerve forces are restored and mental powers are improved. The ability to reason is increased. The powers of attention and association are quickened while memory of past events is often recovered. Dr. Tanner and others even testified to the development of psychic powers during the fast, which Dr. Tanner felt explained "why the old prophets and seers so often resorted to fasting as a means of spiritual illumination."

Fasting thus serves many purposes in terms of physiology and chemistry. It produces rejuvenation of tissues, induces autolysis of abnormal growths, improves the powers of digestion and assimilation, re-establishes normal chemistry and secretion, affords the organs of the body a physiological rest, increases elimination, promotes nerve energy recuperation, strengthens the mind, and perhaps improves function in various ways which we do not yet understand. Obviously these factors are of considerable importance in determining the physical condition of the body. They may mean the difference between strength and weakness, health and disease, and perhaps even life and death.

❧ IV ❧

Efficiency of Fasting

O<small>N THE BASIS</small> of our knowledge regarding the physiological effects of fasting, we are justified in assuming that, theoretically at least, fasting should be a very efficient therapeutic agent. However, important as this is, it is not enough. A measure may be theoretically correct, and have a logical and reasonable basis in all respects, and yet in the treatment of disease it does not fulfill expectations. Thus it is necessary that fasting be given thorough consideration from the standpoint of statistics and available records of its use in the treatment of diseases of all types.

The employment of fasting for therapeutic purposes has been very extensive. There are a number of prominent physicians who can be referred to, each of whom has had experience in conducting thousands of fasts. Among these is Dr. Herbert M. Shelton, who has conducted over 30,000 fasts at his institute ranging in length from a few days to as many months. This record involves more experience with fasting than that of any other living physician, and perhaps also exceeds that of any physician of history. The work of the renowned Dr. William Howard Hay, while director of the great Pocana Haven sanatorium in Mount Pocana, Pa., included the supervision of several thousand fasts. Dr. George S. Weger listed the number of patients who were treated at his sanatorium at approximately 5,000. The experience of Dr. Linda Burfield Hazzard covered nearly 2,500 patients. For decades Dr. John M. Tilden treated patients at his fasting institute in Denver, Colorado, and the large Bergholtz Clinic, in Milwaukee, Wisconsin, founded by Dr. Eugene A. Bergholtz, published the case histories of many of its thousands of fasting patients. Other physicians have likewise been active in this work, each conducting scores, hundreds or thousands of fasts, and they have reported the detailed results of their experiences with fasting.

Most of the patients who have been treated at fasting institutes and sanatoriums had for years suffered from ill health. Many of them tried all other forms of healing—drugs, surgery, manipulation, massage, artificial fever treatments, electrical treatments, autosuggestion, etc.—all to no avail. Finally, as a last resort they decided to try fasting. Heart disease, cancer, ulcers, colitis, asthma, sinusitis, arthritis, tumors, gall bladder infection and other ailments, which are so seldom completely and permanently remedied by orthodox means, were common among the afflictions of the patients.

Yet the percentage of recoveries has been amazingly high —exceeding that resulting from the use of any other therapeutic measure. Many patients, after suffering for years from so-called incurable ailments, have been completely restored to health. All physicians caring for the fasting patients have pointed out the unusual efficiency of the fasting treatment. Dr. Shelton, for instance, has reported that 95 per cent of the patients at his institute have recovered health or claimed benefit, and others who have made lengthy observations of his patients under care do confirm that the treatment is highly effective.

Some of the most important statistics on the subject of fasting come from Dr. James McEachen, who applied fasting in the treatment of 715 cases of disease during the period from August, 1952 to March, 1958. All fasts were carefully supervised under ideal conditions in McEachen's sanatorium near Escondido, California. The only limitation in the efficiency of treatment was that many patients did not have time to fast long enough or often enough to obtain maximum benefit. Yet, in 294 of these cases, there was very great improvement or complete recovery; in 360 cases there was moderate benefit, and for the remaining 61 cases, no improvement at all was noted. Thus the average percentage of improved or remedied cases was 88.4 per cent. On the following chart, the diseases treated by Dr. McEachen are listed, along with the numbers of those responding, and not responding, to care.

Disease	Number of Cases	Cases Improved or Remedied	Cases Not Helped
High Blood Pressure	141	141	0
Colitis	88	77	11
Sinusitis	67	64	3
Anemia	60	52	8
Hemorrhoids	51	48	3
Arthritis	47	39	8
Bronchitis	42	39	3
Kidney Disease	41	36	5
Benign Tumors	38	32	6
Heart Disease	33	29	4
Asthma	29	29	0
Ulcers	23	20	3
Hay Fever	19	17	2
Goiter	11	11	0
Pyorrhea	8	6	2
Gallstones	7	6	1
Cancer	5	5	0
Multiple Sclerosis	4	3	1
Cataract	1	0	1

At Pawling Health Manor, in Hyde Park, New York, fasting has been extensively applied in the care of the sick. Dr. Robert R. Gross, director of the sanatorium, has provided vital statistical data pertaining to this work, covering a time period from August of 1957 to July of 1963. Altogether, Dr. Gross lists 484 complete recoveries, 165 partial recoveries and 31 failures for 680 cases of disease under care. This indicates a recovery rate of 71.2 per cent, a partial recovery rate of 24.2 per cent, and a failure rate of 4.6 per cent. Dr. Gross reported that a considerable number of patients did not remain in the sanatorium long enough to fast a sufficient duration of time or as often as recommended when more than one fast was required. This was considered largely responsible for many of the patients who improved, but did not fully recover, or patients who were not helped at all. The emotional states and cooperation extended by different patients also varied considerably and affected the final outcome of the fasts. In addition, there was not always continued contact with patients long after leaving the sanatorium, so some benefits, which are derived months after the fast, could not be recorded. Taking all of these factors into account, the successes attained were quite remarkable. The important data covering these cases is displayed in full in the chart which follows.

Disease	Number of Cases	Cases Recovered	Cases Improved	Cases Not Helped
High Blood Pressure	54	38	16	0
Arthritis	42	28	10	4
Nasal Catarrh	39	36	2	1
Constipation	36	31	3	2
Hepatitis	36	34	2	0
Goiter	33	18	12	3
Psoriasis	32	18	10	4
Heart Disease	31	18	13	0
Mental Disorders	29	19	10	0
Bronchitis	24	22	1	1
Colitis	23	11	12	0
Hemorrhoids	23	18	5	0
Varicose Veins	23	20	2	1
Hay Fever	22	7	15	0

Disease	Number of Cases	Cases Recovered	Cases Improved	Cases Not Helped
Dyspepsia	21	18	3	0
Pyorrhea	20	8	12	0
Asthma	19	16	0	3
Eczema	18	11	4	3
Benign Tumors	18	14	3	1
Insomnia	17	13	2	2
Ulcers	14	8	4	2
Diabetes	14	12	2	0
Kidney Disease	12	10	2	0
Sinusitis	12	9	3	0
Gallstones	11	6	5	0
Anemia	11	7	4	0
Gonorrhea	8	8	0	0
Poliomyelitis	8	6	2	0
Appendicitis	6	6	0	0
Epilepsy	5	3	2	0
Acne Vulgaris	5	3	2	0
Multiple Sclerosis	4	0	2	2
Tuberculosis	2	2	0	0

Dr. William L. Esser has observed several thousand fasting cases under controlled conditions at his Florida sanitarium. Although detailed data for all of these cases has not been published, Dr. Esser has furnished statistical information pertaining to a sampling of 155 patients, upon which very careful records were kept. Among these patients, a total of 31 different types of disease were treated. These included, among others, ulcers, tumors, tuberculosis, sinusitis, pyorrhea, Parkinson's disease, heart disease, cancer, insomnia, gallstones, epilepsy, colitis, hay fever, bronchitis, asthma and arthritis. The length of the shortest fast was five days; that of the longest fast was 55 days. In many cases the length of the fasts was restricted by time and financial limitations, with only about 20 per cent of the patients remaining in the sanatorium long enough to fast as long as recommended.

Of the 155 patients, 113 were completely restored to health; 31 were partially recovered, and 12 patients were not helped at all. Thus the rate of complete recovery was 71 per cent; of partial recovery, 20 per cent, and of failure, 9 per cent. In view of the character of diseases treated, this represents a very high degree of efficiency, as compared to other therapeutic measures.

Sinclair collected statistics of people who had fasted without professional supervision. In some cases their diseases were diagnosed by physicians but the fasts were usually undertaken on the patients' own initiative. The fasts covered 117 people; the total number of fasts taken was 277, and the average number of days per fast was six. Ninety of the fasts exceeded four days in length, and six were 30 days or longer. Many of the fasts lasted only a few days.

One hundred of the 117 people reported complete recovery or some benefit from fasting, indicating a total percentage of slightly more than 85 per cent who were helped. A total of 116 diseases, of 30 different types, were listed as completely or partially remedied. As some of the people suffered from more than one disease, the number of diseases helped was higher than the number of patients. Of those who were not helped, about half had fasted only a few days and some of the rest gave wrong breaking of the fast as the reason for the failure. The therapeutic record of fasting can be further seen in considering the use of this measure in the treatment of a number of specific diseases.

Prognosis in the case of many eye diseases is good if fasting is employed. Numerous cases of visual defects have been completely remedied by fasting, though some mechanical defects cannot be corrected of course, and certain eye ailments require aid which fasting cannot give. When the muscles of the eyes suffer from a lack of tone, strength, flexibility, suppleness and coordination, special eye exercises will give more benefit than fasting, though fasting may be used to supplement this treatment.

Among the eye conditions for which fasting is often a specific remedy are cataract, congestion of the conjunctiva, catarrhal and granular conjunctivitis, glaucoma, iritis, keratitis and stye. Early cataract generally disappears on the fast; advanced cases may disappear, but recovery is much less certain. Dr. Shelton records one case in which blindness of one eye (due to cataract) completely disappeared on a fast of 18 days. Dr. Gerald Benesh reports equal success in treating a complete cataract, which yielded to a 21 day fast. The forms of conjunctivitis require only cleanliness and fasting for recovery, with short fasts in acute cases and long fasts in chronic cases. When glaucoma exists, the hardness of the eye tends to disappear, with the excessive fluid being absorbed, on fasts of two or three weeks in duration. In advanced cases, when complete atrophy is present, the prognosis is not favorable, with blindness the usual result. Iritis, keratitis and stye need only fasting, cleanliness and rest, with recovery the general rule unless previous suppressive treatment leaves permanent damage to sight.

Respiratory ailments respond quickly to the fast. Hay fever improves in virtually all cases without any change of climate. Patients with catarrh recover on the fast, although eliminations may increase temporarily on the early days of the fast. Polyps, which may be present, are absorbed; the thickened membranes return to their normal thickness, though the atrophied structures of advanced catarrh cannot be rebuilt. Sinusitis responds readily to the fast; only a few days of fasting will bring relief in some cases; in others long fasts may be necessary. Chronic laryngitis yields quickly to the fast. Chronic cases of asthma usually attain much relief within just a few days of fasting, with complete recovery in a matter of weeks. Those asthmatics who are unable to sleep lying in bed and consequently sleep in a sitting position are usually relieved sufficiently within 36 hours without food to sleep in bed. Dr. Benesh refers to different patients recovering from severe and long-standing asthma on fasts of different duration. One case required two fasts of 15 and 21 days; another responded to several short fasts of 2, 5, 6 and 7 days; the third fasted 26 days, and two fasts of 23 and 26 days were necessary in the most advanced case. Of the hundreds of asthmatics treated by Dr. Shelton with fasting, only three failed to recover. Congestion of the lungs is rapidly and safely remedied in all cases through fasting, and bronchitis responds equally well to treatment. The most important respiratory disease, tuberculosis of the lungs, has often been treated with the fast. In the vast majority of cases the prognosis is very favorable. While fasting, the tubercular cough usually becomes very mild or altogether disappears. In some cases much improvement occurs on the fast, followed by complete recovery during a period of proper nutrition with adequate fresh air and careful exposure to sunlight. A short fasting period is usually given preference in tuberculosis cases because of the difficulty some patients have had in gaining weight after long fasts. Yet, a number of patients have recovered during long fasts and then rapidly returned to normal weight. It is possible that the difficulties which occurred in other cases were due to poor control of the dietary after fasting.

Various forms of goiter have been helped by fasting. When simple goiter exists, the enlargement tends to subside to normal during the course of the fast. If the disease has reached the stage where the soft goiter becomes a form of tumor, called an adenoma, improvement or recovery is still possible without surgery, although a longer period of abstinence may be required. Even when the goiter displays rapidly developing evidences of toxicity, as in exophthalmic goiter, there is positive hope for the patient. Dr. Weger stated that "almost without exception, ex-

ard Geithner, of the Blaubeuren Sanatorium in Germany, reported that three multiple sclerosis patients "who agreed to the fasting-cure were free of paralysis after 18 to 21 days of fasting." One of these patients had a new episode of paralysis after the fast, which, in turn, was cured by another fast of 14 days. During the following three years of observation, there was no recurrence of paralysis.

Literally thousands of abnormal growths have undergone dissolution and absorption on fasts. Shelton, Hazzard, Tilden and Rabagliati, among others, report many such cases. Armstrong, of England, declared that he had "seen lumps in female breasts, treated to a fast, some after diagnosis by experts, the bulk after self-diagnosis, and to disappear, on water only, in from four to twenty days." Macfadden remarked that his experience had shown "beyond all possible doubt that a foreign growth of any kind can be absorbed into the circulation by simply compelling the body to use every unnecessary element contained within it for food."

Whereas most abnormal growths that have disappeared while fasting have been benign tumors, a considerable number have also been diagnosed as malignant. Dr. Shelton states that he has seen cancer patients "become free from all pain in twenty-four hours to three days when the drugging was discontinued and all feeding stopped." He also reported actual recovery of one case which had previously been diagnosed as cancer in as little as three days of fasting. Of course longer fasts are required in most instances of suspected cancer, and Dr. Hazzard recorded a case in which 45 days of fasting were required before recovery was complete. Another experienced worker in this field, Dr. Rasmus Alsaker, supervised "the return to health of many individuals diagnosed as having cancer of the stomach" with the fasting treatment, although he did not discount the possibility of mistakes of diagnosis in these cases.

As a rule the chances of recovery from cancer depend largely upon the stage of the disease and the history of previous therapeutic treatment. In early cancer, which has not been treated with surgery nor radiation, and which has not involved the prolonged use of pain-killing drugs, the prognosis is frequently favorable. The slow absorption of the neoplasm of cancer can then be expected in many cases. In certain cases there is not complete absorption, though further growth may be checked. If the neoplasm of cancer has been broken with exploratory or therapeutic surgery, with release of cancer cells to other parts of the body, and if tissues have been weakened with extensive X-ray therapy, the chances of recovery are markedly lower. If, in addition to these adverse factors, the patient has been kept under a state of sedation until he is suffering more from the effects of drug addiction than cancer, we find the least favorable prognosis. However, even when cancer is in its hopeless stage, fasting may be considered of some value in reducing pain and bringing the patient to a more comfortable end than could otherwise occur.

Fasting is of exceptional value in the treatment of appendicitis. Recovery generally takes places within a few days to two weeks of fasting. The advantage of fasting over surgery in such cases, especially those which are most severe, is seen by the fact that the mortality rate in cases of acute, gangrenous, ruptured appendicitis with peritonitis is only 1.43 per cent when the operation is deferred. Immediate operations for the same condition have provided a mortality rate of 10.64 per cent (Reference: Journal of the American Medical Association, Dec. 5, 1936, page 1910). Further, the average death rate in all forms of appendicitis when surgery is resorted to is 2.3 per cent, with 16,000 of an average of 520,000 patients dying annually in the United States. The efficiency of fasting in such cases is shown by the experience of Dr. Hay, who treated over 400 patients who were afflicted with acute and chronic appendicitis. In nineteen cases the appendix had already ruptured. Yet complete recovery occurred in every case without a single failure or fatality. In no instance was surgery resorted to. Each patient was fasted until recovery was complete.

Fasting has been used with success in the treatment of various forms of sexual disorders and venereal diseases. Dr. Hazzard points out that the bacillus of gonorrhea "cannot long exist if the products of elimination are normal, and if cleanliness, especially of the female, is properly observed." She states that the "irritating symptoms of local venereal infection yield to treatment (fasting) in a few days, and convalescence brings no supervening annoyance as expressed in urethral stricture, prostatic congestion, etc."

Regarding syphilis, Dr. Shew wrote that "The hunger-cure is nowhere more applicable." The great medical authority, Dr. Robert Bartholow, also pointed out the value of fasting in such cases. Dr. Shelton states that "without exception" his patients with syphilis "have gotten well in four to eight weeks under hygienic care." Dr. Tilden refers to recovery from syphilis "in from six weeks to two months without aftermaths of any kind" when the fasting treatment, followed by correct diet, is employed. Dr. Weger claims that the "local lesions of the first-stage heal with startling rapidity," and that "pharyngeal, labial, and buccal ulcerations frequently disappear before the tenth day of fasting."

In treating diseases of the female reproductive system, fasting relieves congestion, removes infection, relaxes tissues and restores tone to the affected area. Abnormal growths of the womb tend to be partially or completely absorbed during the fast. The supposed need for surgical operation, with its attendant dangers and disadvantages, is thus reduced or eliminated when diseases of the female organs occur. In such simple conditions as painful and excessive menstruation, fasting is also of distinct value. Dr. Hazzard stated that "From one to three day's abstinence from food will correct excessive menstruation, and, when no mechanical defect is present relief is obtained within twenty-four hours when the flow is accompanied by pain."

Diabetes was first treated with fasting by the famous French clinician, A. Guelpa, of Paris. Dr. Guelpa noted that fasting for three or four successive days rendered the urine of the patient with severe diabetes sugar-free, and effected pronounced improvement in the state of health, with no aggravation of the disease in any case. The American physician, Dr. Heinrich Stern, was next to treat diabetes with fasting and reduced nutritional intake, and his many hundreds of patients as a rule responded favorably. Dr. Stern found that, though there were certain cases of the severest types of diabetes "which no amount of fasting would render sugar-free," the majority of patients "cease to excrete sugar within forty-eight to sixty hours," with an occasional patient fasting six days or longer before the glycosuric symptom disappeared. In approximately seventy-five per cent of all cases the urine was also rendered free from ketones, though this required a longer period of fasting. Dr. Frederick Allen, of the Rockefeller Institute, has also employed the "starvation treatment" of diabetes, and his important work with fasting and restricted diet in 1915 effected a 60 per cent reduction in deaths from diabetic coma.

Also treated in many instances by fasting is the serious disease, epilepsy. Several decades ago Dr. Rabagliati noted that fasting "seems to be of very great efficacy in the treatment of epilepsy." In 1932 Dr. C. Clemmessen came to a similar conclusion as a result of his work at the Hospital for Nervous and Mental Diseases in Dianlund, Denmark. On the basis of 155 fasting treatments for epilepsy, Dr. Clemmessen found that in the great majority of cases, fasting caused the epileptic attacks to cease within four to five days, irrespective of the previous duration of illness. Fasting was equally effective whether the epilepsy was of organic nature or cryptogenetic, and it seemed to be most effective in cases with very frequent seizures.

Dr. Alsaker stated that "It is a revelation to some persons who fast how clearly the mind can function." This being true, it might be expected that various forms of insanity would be helped by fasting. Widespread experience by many physicians has shown that fasting is not only valuable in caring for the insane patient but that it frequently succeeds where all other forms of treatment have failed. Fasting can not only be applied in promoting absorbtion of brain tumors and improving the physical condition of the brain and nervous system; it also has been used successfully in treating mental aberrations which were thought to have purely emotional causes.

Of those fasting practitioners who have cared for mental patients, Dr. Hay had some of the most notable experiences. He applied the absolute fast and partial fast, along with proper nutrition, and he reported excellent results in the majority of cases. Of seventeen cases of dementia praecox brought to Dr. Hay, five cases were unmanageable without restraint but all others were carefully treated and "made splendid comebacks" to a high grade of mental health. Dr Hay described one mental patient who "was wholly irrational, could not even answer questions, having both amnesic and ataxic asphasia, cried continually, and required a special nurse to restrain her from throwing herself out of the window." Yet after ten days of partial fasting, utilizing only the extracted juices of fruits and vegetables, followed by 20 days of controlled diet, the patient returned to her home "as sane as she had ever been before in her life, and a very bright young woman."

Fasting is the safest and most appropriate method of treating varicose veins. It does not destroy or coagulate the veins, which are accomplished by other methods at the cost of overworking the deeper blood vessels, but it does heal varicose ulcers, helps to restore tonicity to the walls of the veins, reduces their size and provides freedom from pain. In young people who are affected by varicosities of small to moderate size, full recovery is usually possible. For the patient past middle age, with severe varicosities, definite improvement with comfort may be expected but complete recovery is rare. In all cases, proper nutrition and adequate exercise after the fast are necessary to prevent excess fluid in the tissues and assure continued improvement or maintenance of normal tone of the walls of the veins.

When varicosities occur in the vein near the anus, as in hemorrhoids, fasting is also of much assistance. During the fast, there is little or no bowel action to occasion further irritation, and healing of the affected areas is permitted. As early as 1854 Dr. Joel Shew, in discussing "The Hunger-Cure," stated that "There is nothing in the world that will produce so great relief in hemorrhoids as fasting." In cases "where to evacuate the bowels would put the patient into an agony, amounting almost to spasms," there was marked improvement after only three or four days of fasting. Dr. McCoy described one case history of hemorrhoids in which the patient was unable to walk for several days before the fast because of the severe pain that persisted day and night. Yet after only ten days of fasting "all signs of the hemorrhoids had disappeared, and the rectum seemed to be in quite a normal condition." While writing on this same subject, Carrington stated: "I may add that I have observed some most striking examples of such cures myself."

Arthritis, rheumatism and gout as a rule respond quickly to the fast. Most patients experience freedom from severe arthritic pains within a few days after the fast is instituted. There is gradual disappearance of the swelling and complete or partial absorption of the deformity by autolysis providing complete ossification of the joint is not present. Dr. Casey A. Wood, Professor of Chemistry in the Medical Dept. of Bishop's College in Montreal, issued a report concerning seven case histories of acute articular rheumatism. These patients were speedily restored to health during four to eight days of fasting. Dr. Wood also mentioned forty other similar cases from his own private practice in which recovery from this disease was achieved, and in no instance was it necessary to fast longer than ten days. However, patients affected by severe chronic arthritis of long standing must usually undertake longer fasts. Those who are so badly crippled that they are unable to walk alone, comb their hair or even feed themselves usually achieve restoration of considerable motion to the stiffened joints during a single fast, although complete recovery (when this is possible) in some of these cases may require a second fast.

Simple gall bladder and bile duct infection is completely remedied during fasts of short to moderate duration. The pus is removed, the inflammation subsides and the tissues are healed during this physiological rest. When stones have formed in the gall bladder, somewhat longer fasts may be required but recovery is to be expected. The patient with gallstones finds relief from severe pain after the first few days of the fast, although complete recovery in the more advanced cases may require up to 20 to 25 days of abstinence from food. During the fast, the stones soften, later disintegrate and then pass through the bile duct into the small intestine. Some pain may occur during the passage of stones but this does not involve the extreme discomfort frequently experienced prior to the fast.

Fasting is without doubt the most rapid and effective method of remedying high blood pressure. Indeed, hundreds of consecutive patients have been treated for this condition without a single complete failure. Even patients who have failed to respond to all of the customary treatment of high blood pressure do respond to fasting. Shelton has reported one case in which a systolic pressure of 295 was brought down to 115 during three weeks of fasting. And the cures in these cases tend to be lasting. If the blood pressure falls below normal during the fast, it will rise to normal later, but actual hypertension does not redevelop so long as good nutritional habits are maintained after the fast.

Heart disease has been treated by fasting in a very large number of cases. Fortunately the most common causes of heart trouble—narrowing of the coronary artery and formation of thrombus in this artery—are usually corrected by fasting. As a rule the thrombus and excess fatty material lining the walls of the artery are absorbed by autolysis during the course of the fast. Other heart diseases, such as acute myocarditis, fatty overgrowth of the heart, endocarditis and ordinary pericarditis, also respond very favorably to fasting. Two less common heart conditions, hemopericardium and calcified pericardium, can usually be remedied only partially when any form of help is possible.

Of the one hundred and more pathological conditions which affect the skin, most can be treated successfully with fasting. Even in so serious a condition as leprosy, the skin ulcerations and nodules have disappeared in just a few weeks of fasting and sunbathing. For simple acne and other common skin diseases, recovery tends to be more rapid, with most cases responding to care in one to two weeks or less. Eczema and severe skin diseases, however, may require longer fasts. In all cases, improvement is limited to the removal of swelling, inflamation, excess scaly tissue, ulcerations, etc. For this reason early treatment in many cases is recommended. Once severe scar tissue has formed, little or nothing can be done to restore the original skin texture.

In particular it is true that fasting is of extraordinary value in the treatment of all acute diseases. Regardless of the forms such ailments have taken, fasting has been employed as the first requirement and continued until the acute symptoms subsided. Not only is recovery much more rapid than when the customary treatments are given, but the mortality rate is much lower than usual. Indeed, some fasting practitioners report no mortality rate at all for the acutely-ill, and Dr. Shelton states that, of the hundreds of such patients he has cared for, "not a single one" has "died or failed to recover" or developed complications of any kind.

Typhoid fever patients recover in about two weeks while fasting, in absence of most of the distressing symptoms which result from feeding and giving medication to such patients. Smallpox takes only the form of a light disease when fasting is instituted immediately. There is only very slight itching, no complications, and very rarely any pitting at all. In cases of scarlet fever, the rash disappears within four to seven days and the fever is gone by the fourth day. Mumps disappear within six to ten days of fasting, with no danger of complications. Regarding rheumatic fever, Dr. Weger claims that "in no case in which food was withheld from the onset did the temperature remain above normal for longer than ten days, and recovery was prompt without merging into the sub-acute and chronic stage." In the case of influenza, Dr. Weger points to the "rapid decline of all symptoms and abatement of temperature usually within three days," while fasting, with no mortality rate at all. Erysipelas, he declares, is "readily checked without pursuing its usual round-trip course." Fever disappears on the third or fourth day, with no abscesses or secondary infections. Dr. Weger not only refers to recovery from malaria "in all stages," but states that no relapses "have been reported on return from fever-infested surroundings."

There are no age barriers to fasting. Both aged individuals and young children have fasted with great benefit. Even infants may be placed on short fasts, and there is one record of a 2-year-old child fasting to recovery from poliomyelitis, with paralysis, on a 47-day fast, during which time the weight fell from 32 pounds to 15 pounds. Obviously such long fasts in children are the exception rather than the general rule, and they are not always to be recommended. Nor is long fasting often necessary during childhood, most children's diseases disappearing rapidly during short facts.

The only periods of life in which the use of fasting may be questioned are those of lactation and pregnancy. Fasting stops the secretion of milk and hence prevents the mother from nursing her child. During pregnancy long fasts to remedy chronic diseases are certainly inadvisable, though when acute disease exists, there may be a short fast until most or all of the symptoms subside.

Clearly, in terms of strict efficiency, fasting is of exceptional value as a therapeutic measure. It is in no sense a cure-all, nor is it the only method whereby health can be restored. As was noted, some conditions in their advanced stages do not always recover on the fast. Further, the same results which often occur while fasting may occur by employing certain diets, though the latter method frequently is much less certain and incomparably slower than the fast. For speed and certainty in recovery the fast has no equal in the cases of most diseases, as the employment of fasting in thousands of cases has clearly shown. As regards efficiency, it is in a class by itself.

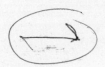

V

The Complete Fast

IT IS THE COMMON and popular opinion that fasting and starvation are synonymous. Upon first hearing of therapeutic fasting, many speak of it as the "starvation cure." Actually, there is an important difference between fasting and starvation, and though both imply abstinence from food, the physiological effects are in no sense similar.

When food is consumed at regular intervals, the body stores sufficient quantities of nutritive matter to last for a considerable period of time during later periods of abstinence. From the start of every fast, the body commences to nourish and feed itself upon such reserves. The cells accordingly diminish in size and there are changes in the colloidal condition of the protoplasm. Cell proliferation itself continues. The chief weight losses consist of fat, muscle, tissue, blood and water. Such vital body parts as the brain, spinal cord, nerves, teeth and bones are well sustained on the fast with practically no losses. In children the skeletal structure continues to grow, the marrow being drawn upon for nourishment for this purpose.

Such is the nutritive aspect of fasting. The body continues to receive, from its reserves, the sustaining materials of life. There is of course a limit to this supply. When all normal food reserves have been exhausted the body must derive other means of nourishment. It then enters a period of true starvation and feeds upon the vital tissues and hitherto unchanged body parts.

This is the stage which Prof. Morgulis states "is character-ized by the predominance of pathological phenomena caused by the prolonged stringency of nourishment and exhaustion of tissues." Morgulis further points out that "the morphologi-cal changes observed in advanced starvation are practically identical with those found in every pathological condition and present nothing peculiar." During this period the healthy tis-sues are wasted, the vitality is depleted, and the body is emaciated. The blood atrophies; the cells of the liver, heart, kidneys, pancreas and other organs become the seat of degen-erative processes. As the conditions reach their advanced stages, death occurs.

Fasting begins with the omission of the first meal and ends with the exhaustion of all food reserves. Starvation begins at this time and ends with death. Thus where the one process ends, the other begins. Whereas scientific fasting is accom-panied by beneficial results, the elimination of pathology, and rejuvenation, starvation is accompanied by the develop-ment of pathology, degeneration, and the most disastrous consequences.

When the food reserves of the body have been consumed, certain symptoms occur which indicate the end of the fasting period. There is invariably a return of hunger and a removal of coating from the tongue. The edges and tip of the tongue clear first, with the rest quickly following. The bad taste in the mouth and the offensive breath likewise disappear at this time. The pulse and temperature, which may have been abnormal, become normal. The eyes frequently brighten, sali-vary secretion is normalized, and the urine, which may have been discolored, becomes clear. Of these symptoms, the return of hunger and clearing of the tongue are the most important, and are regarded by some as the only certain and unmistak-able signs which denote the completion of the fast. The others are usually present also, but it is the return of hunger and the condition of the tongue which are regarded as the determining factors.

The return of hunger and the clean tongue do not always arrive at exactly the same time. One may arrive a few hours or more before the other. Under any conditions the fast should be broken at the appearance of either symptom. One should not, for instance, hesitate to break the fast if there is an unmistakable desire for food even though the tongue is not clean, and vice versa. In those very rare cases in which hunger is not lost on the fast, the clearing of the tongue will suffice as a guide in determining the completion of the fast.

Dr. Hereward Carrington describes the feelings of the fasting patient at the completion of the fasting period in these words: "A sudden and complete rejuvenation; a feeling of lightness, buoyancy, and good health steals over the patient in an irresistible way, bringing contentment and a general feeling of well being, and the possession of a superabundance of animal spirits."

Recognition of the great difference between fasting and starvation, and the symptoms which denote the end of one period and the beginning of the other, is of vital importance in the employment of therapeutic fasting. Abstinence from food can be exceedingly dangerous if one attempts to set in advance the length of a period of fasting without regard to the differences between the two phases of inanition. On the other hand, an understanding of these points eliminates all danger of true starvation. The symptoms which indicate the end of the fasting period are easily recognizable in all cases, and the simple knowledge of what these are can be of assurance to both the physician and layman that the fast will not be extended too long.

The fast which lasts to the return of hunger and the consequent end of the fasting period is said to be "complete." It has carried the work of renovation, rejuvenation and cleansing to its final consummation. The patient has then undergone the most thorough therapeutic treatment that is possible to provide. His body has lost most or all of its superfluous materials, waste matter and diseased or dead tissues. It is then in

an ideal condition upon which to build new healthy protoplasm, with consequent vigorous health.

The time required for the fast to reach completion varies
in the individual cases. Some have exhausted their food reserves after as little as 20 per cent of the body weight was lost,
with others remaining in the fasting period when over half
—even up to 60 per cent—of the body tissues were consumed.
It is easily understood, of course, that the overweight individual can fast longer than one who is thin. Among those who
are particularly obese, the extra layers of fat and other tissue
will provide the body with nourishment long after the normal
patient would reach the termination of the fasting period.

Measuring the fast in terms of days, weeks and months, we
find that some patients have fasted as long as ninety days
before experiencing the return of hunger and other symptoms
denoting the end of the fast. Sinclair reported what was perhaps the shortest complete fast on record, that of his wife, in
which case the tongue rapidly cleared after only ten days of
abstinence from food. For most patients, however, the completion of the fasting period is not reached at such extremes.
Though exact statistics listing the length of the average complete fast are not available, an estimate of from four to seven
weeks is probably fairly close.

A number of physicians have maintained that every fast
should be carried to completion, unless adverse symptoms
force other action. Among these were Dewey, Carrington and
Hazzard. Dr. Dewey mentioned cases in which the patients
broke their fasts prematurely and were unable to digest the
foods, vomiting everything that was eaten. Upon resumption
of fasting, and continuance to the return of hunger, normal
digestive powers were restored and foods could be handled
with ease. Dr. Carrington referred to the artificial breaking of
a fast before the return of hunger as "an abomination, and an
outrage upon the system which cannot be too strongly depre-
cated." Dr. Hazzard believed that "Not until hunger indicates

the need for food is the organism in condition to receive and transform it into tissue structure."

Today the majority of practitioners accept, with reservations, the advisability of carrying the fast to its natural termination. The complete fast is looked upon as an ideal, but seldom as a necessity. Cases in which digestion was difficult or impossible before the fast was "complete" were common in the Dewey-Carrington era of fasting because many fasts were then broken on solid foods. Today such cases are rare, and most practicing physicians have not encountered them, simply because of the advance of knowledge pertaining to the proper method of breaking the fast. If the correct liquid foods are given, a fast for chronic disease can be broken at almost any time without trouble. When acute disease is present, digestion is often impossible for a time and the fast must continue, though this is due to the disease itself rather than the fast.

Certainly it is true that the utmost benefit is derived from a complete fast. In the case of some severe degenerative diseases recovery is impossible without such a fast, and in rare instances one complete fast may not even be sufficient, with fasting again being resumed after a long period of eating to rebuild the food reserves of the body. For the majority of acute diseases, on the other hand, a complete fast is very seldom necessary, with recovery usually taking place long before the termination of the fasting period is reached. For chronic diseases in their early stages, a short fast of a week or two often gives the desired results. When the patient is very weak or emaciated, certainly a complete fast is not called for.

It is apparent that no strict rule applying to all patients and diseases can be applied here. The length of each fast must be determined individually; it cannot safely and effectively be called in advance. All that can first be given is a general estimate; as the fast progresses and the symptoms subside, the correct time to give food can be chosen. For those whose condition and circumstances are most favorable, the fast can perhaps be carried to completion if this is so desired. For others

—no doubt the majority—this will be considered neither necessary nor desirable. Each physician or individual must give judgment in these cases as he sees fit. The problem is not a difficult one; with adequate knowledge, observation and care, the fast may be broken at the most opportune time, without danger, and with the possible benefits and objects in view having been secured.

❧ VI ❧

Safety of the Fast

WHILE RECOGNIZING the value of fasting as a specific remedy for certain diseases, it is also necessary to consider the question of safety. It is one thing to be given the possibility or probability of recovery; it is another to be given this without any attendant danger, with assurance that a gamble is not being made which may involve disadvantages as well as advantages. A valuable therapeutic measure should both provide good results in treating disease and at the same time be associated with a minimum of danger. In the case of many therapeutic measures this requirement is not met, and one disease is being cured, while perhaps more serious ones are being created through the toxic influences of drugs or the loss of important organs through surgery. It is important to understand the position of fasting in these respects.

Generally speaking, initial consideration of fasting is associated with fear both of death and the possibility of doing serious harm to the body. On the surface, at least, such fear may have a logical and reasonable basis, considering the fact that tradition has provided the almost universal impression that just a week or two of abstinence is associated with grave danger and possible death. This has led to analysis of fasting by many physicians who considered any observations of actual fasting to be completely out of the question. The conclusions thus drawn inevitably were completely theoretical and speculative, there being no actual cases of fasting present upon which practical deductions could have been made.

Unfortunately reports of fasting all too frequently are founded upon the very basis mentioned, with the result that objections to fasting have been made which, though they may sound logical from the theoretical evidence at hand, are completely fantastic to those who have done either laboratory or therapeutic work with fasting. In consequence statements have been made that fasting weakens the heart, causes the heart to collapse, causes the stomach to atrophy or makes the digestive juices digest the stomach, produces deficiency disease, causes the teeth to decay, lowers the resistance of the body to disease, causes degeneration of cells, is opposed to our natural instincts, causes edema, causes acidosis, and last but not least, creates a grave danger of death.

In actual experience not a single one of these objections to fasting has been found to have any basis in fact. Quite apart from being weakened or collapsed by fasting, the heart is given a rest and thus allowed to gain new strength. Serious cases of heart disease have actually recovered while fasting. The stomach, in fact the entire digestive tract, is strengthened by fasting. There is no atrophy or impairment whatsoever. Patients who have always suffered from digestive weakness fully recover while fasting.

As for deficiency diseases—these do not occur while fasting. Beliefs to the contrary have resulted from studies of deficient diets. As a result, nutritionists speak of the "probable appearance of deficiency disease" on long fasts. It is assumed that if diets lacking sufficient minerals and vitamins produce deficiency diseases, a fast, which supplies no additional minerals and vitamins, must do likewise. During a fast, when the body's energy is not used in the work of digestion and assimilation, the need for minerals is lowered. The reserves of these elements in the body are sufficient to meet all needs. It is for this reason that no deficiency diseases, including dental decay, occur on the fast, though they often follow a diet of refined foods. Man can live much longer on water alone than he can on a diet of white flour and water simply because use of the flour increases the need for other elements to enable the body to digest, assimilate and metabolize the flour. Hence, not one, but many, severe deficiency diseases quickly arise on such a diet. Deficiency diseases frequently even recover on the fast, due to better assimilation of elements already stored in the body. In this connection, the contrast between deficiency diets and fasting is pointed out by Prof. Morgulis, who states that "our observation that the chronically underfed dog became debilitated in a measure not commonly noted in animals which undergo a straight fast is also borne out by more extensive study of this matter by Benedict, Miles, Roth and Smith."

Claims that fasting causes degeneration of cells result from studies of animals in the last stages of starvation. Kellogg, for instance, refers to the work of Statkewitsch, who found that prolonged fasting in many animals was associated with degeneration. Not distinguishing between the periods of fasting and starvation thus leads to wrong impressions. Rejuvenation rather than degeneration is the result of fasting.

Quite apart from lowering resistance to disease, and producing diseases such as tuberculosis, which are believed to follow low resistance, fasting increases the resistance to disease and has been used successfully as a specific remedy of tuberculosis. Resistance depends upon chemical balance, abundant nerve force and all of the physiological conditions which fasting produces. The numerous complete recoveries from disease which occur while fasting are in themselves evidence that the power to overcome infection is raised on the fast, rather than susceptibility increased.

Animal experiments substantiate these points. Roger and Jause found that fasting produces an increased tolerance toward bacilli coli in rabbits. Three to eleven days after the animals had fasted for five to seven days, the inoculation of bacterial culture took place. Without exception all control rabbits developed the infection, whereas the rabbits which had been fasted escaped all symptoms of infection.

Though instinct is not given as a scientific reason for fasting or anything else, it is only fair to point out that fasting is not opposed to our natural instincts in the sense that is often reported. It is said that to fast is to thwart our normal sensations of hunger. The implication here is that hunger is normal throughout the fast, whereas the fact is that it only exists for the first few days, and when acute disease is present, it often does not exist at all. Unquestionably the customary practice of forced feeding in the case of acute disease is opposed to our natural instincts. Even among wild and domestic animals fasting appears to be an instinctive practice. In case of an occasional illness, or a serious wound resulting from accident or battle, they frequently fast until recovery is well under way or complete.

Beliefs that fasting produces edema have resulted from the misuse of fasting. Frederick Hoelzel writes that he has "not known of any case of fasting, even when for only days, where some post-fasting edema was not present." In Mr. Hoelzel's experience, cotton fibre, lemon juice, and salt were given as food after fasting. It is quite surprising that the aftereffects were not more serious than actually occurred. The development of edema under such a regime, with liberal amounts of water, is to be expected. On salt-water fasts, or when salt is used liberally with water immediately after fasts, the tissues become water-logged, as the body attempts to protect itself from the irritating effects of the salt by holding it in solution, even though this calls for an excess of water in the tissues. The objection here is to salt, not fasting. In the general use of fasting, no salt-water is ever used, and edema has not developed, except in very rare instances when the fasts were broken on incorrect food or when excessive amounts of food were ingested immediately after fasting, practices which of course are avoided by all physicians experienced with fasting. It may be added here that fasting is frequently used as a remedy for edema, and results have proven very satisfactory. Quite apart from causing the ailment, it is the most effective means of causing its disappearance.

It is true that blood alkalinity is slightly lowered during the fast. However, this never reaches the point that true "acidosis" exists. There are always sufficient alkaline reserves in the body to prevent this condition. In all cases the blood is rapidly restored to its normal alkalinity when eating is resumed, and there is no evidence to indicate that the slightly lowered alkalinity during the fast has any detrimental effects.

The mortality rate of patients who fast is extremely low. It is true, of course, that in rare instances people have died while fasting, though this cannot rightly be ascribed to the fast unless improper care was taken of the fasting patient or the fast was broken on improper food. The fact is that there is no record of death from a properly conducted fast. Deaths while fasting are generally due to the presence of organic disease. Of the 2,500 fasting patients of Dr. Linda Burfield Hazzard, eighteen died, indicating a mortality rate of only seven-tenths of one percent. In the case of each death an autopsy was performed, and in no instance was the death found due to fasting. In each case the medical examiners gave the presence of organic disease as the cause of death.

It must be remembered that people who have fasted usually were victims of the most serious diseases. Most of them tried many forms of other medical and drugless treatment before ever considering fasting. It is generally at a last resort that the fasting method is employed. Many are near death when they start the fast. It is obvious that, under such conditions, some of the patients will die whether they fast or not. The development of pathology has simply gone too far, and nothing, not even fasting, can always prevent death in such cases. Actually the percentage of deaths while fasting is unquestionably much lower than is the case when the same diseases are treated by the usual orthodox means.

In terms of safety, fasting is without doubt one of the best and most practical therapeutic agents. There are virtually no contradictions in fasting, in the sense that one part of the body is helped while another is harmed. In this respect it differs from so many other methods of treatment, which suppress one symptom, only to create others. Fasting helps the diseased organ in the same sense that it helps all other organs and tissues. Thus in securing a remedy for one disease, the body is made less liable to be afflicted by others. Health is restored by the safest and most effective means.

❧ VII ❧

Symptoms of the Fast

FASTING INVOLVES a continual physiological change in
the body. Rejuvenescence, autolysis, increased assimilation, elimination and other processes are taking place. Under
these conditions it is to be expected that there will be outward
manifestations of the changes occurring in the body. Such
manifestations may be either pleasant or discomforting,
more often the latter, and, though in no sense a cause for
concern, they should be understood and expected.

During the first day of the fast, a marked desire for food is
usually present by afternoon or evening. On the second day
the desire is often greatly increased, with the degree of hunger reaching its climax. On the third day the hunger usually
abates and in some cases it entirely disappears. In nearly all
cases the disappearance of hunger is complete by the fourth
or fifth day. From this time onward there is not only no desire
for food, but marked repugnance for food. Nausea and vomiting can even occur at the sight and smell of food. This state
continues until natural hunger returns weeks or months later,
or until the fast is broken, when appetite rapidly returns. Dr.
Weger reported that about one in each forty of his patients
failed to lose their hunger on the fast. Other physicians also
reported similar experiences. No reason is known to account
for this abnormal reaction, and though it in no way dimin-
ishes the effectiveness of the fast, it does make fasting rather
difficult. Fortunately such cases are the exception rather than
the general rule.

The tongue usually becomes heavily coated, and the breath very offensive, within the first few days of fasting. Here too there are very rare exceptions. Dr. Shelton reports three cases in his experience in which the tongue remained clean throughout the fast. Patients have also been observed who exhibited a clean and sweet breath while fasting. In the usual cases, when the reactions of the tongue and breath are normal, the tongue gradually becomes clean, and the breath sweet, as the hunger returns toward the end of the fast, or when the fast is broken. Both of these symptoms while fasting appear to be manifestations of the increased elimination within the body.

The reactions of body temperature vary to some degree with different fasting patients. When there is acute disease, with fever, the temperature gradually drops to normal during the fast. When the temperature is below normal at the beginning of the fast, as is often the case when chronic disease is present, it gradually rises to normal and remains there, although the rate of rise is not always the same, with some patients fasting two, three or more weeks before the rise is to be noted. In rare cases, when no acute disease exists, the temperature rises above normal for short periods. A rapid fall in body temperature has been recorded in a few instances during the very last stages of fasting. Such reaction calls for immediate breaking of the fast and the application of external heat. As a rule the rapid fall in body temperature is a symptom of only the starvation period, marking the complete exhaustion of the body's food reserves. Among animals in the starvation period, the temperature falls rapidly for two to six days before death.

Even though body temperature may be normal while fasting, there is occasionally a slight tendency towards chilliness. This is presumably due to decreased cutaneous circulation, and requires additional clothing or bed covering. The feet often become cold, and in such cases a hot water bottle may be applied to maintain comfort during sleep.

There is usually some variation in the pulse rate during the fast. In some cases it has risen as high as 120, and Macfadden records one case in which it dropped to 20. In most cases of chronic disease, the pulse rises slightly at first, then falls to about 40 or slightly more, after which it rises again to about 60. When there is a disease of the heart present, the pulse rate often varies considerably from the standard. An erratic pulse is quite frequent while fasting. Only when there is a persistent very erratic pulse, or when the pulse remains very high or very low for long periods should the fast be broken. The usual variations and short periods of erratic pulse should be taken for granted.

Most fasting patients sleep less than usual. In some instances no more than three or four hours a day are spent sleeping. Others, especially those who have previously suffered from insomnia, sleep longer during the fast, with insomnia patients having slept as much as 20 out of each 24 hours in some cases.

During the first few weeks of fasting there is occasionally an actual increase in strength. Prof. Luciani found that his fasting subject, Succi, registered a stronger grip on the dynamometer on the twenty-first day of the fast than when it began, and he further stated that the fatigue curve obtained by Succi was the same on the twenty-ninth day of the fast as is obtained from individuals under normal conditions. Dynamometric tests taken of Agnostino Levanzin, on his experimental thirty-one day fast at the Nutrition Laboratory of the Carnegie Institute, showed no decrease in strength. The onetime famous boxers, heavyweight Harry Wills and lightweight Freddy Welsh, both used short fasts during their training periods. In 1913 Macfadden supervised seven days of fasting of athletes who then appeared on the eighth day at Madison Square Garden to perform athletic feats, primarily weight-lifting, which would have been exceptional for even the best athletes while eating. In was on this occasion that Gilbert Low, after breaking his fast at the end of the eighth day, established nine world records for strength and endurance.

An increase in strength is especially noticeable for those who are very weak at the beginning of the fast. Patients have been carried into fasting institutions on stretchers and gained strength so rapidly while fasting that they were walking about again within a few weeks. Macfadden, Carrington, Shelton and others have reported increases in strength among their fasting patients. As a rule they have found that in these cases the increase in strength generally lasts to about three weeks, after which there is a gradual lessening of strength.

Though cases such as have been mentioned are frequent occurrences on the fast, there are many, perhaps the majority, of fasting patients who gradually lose strength from the beginning of the fast to the very end. There are others who maintain strength while fasting, as shown in tests, but who feel weak and languid when not exercising. This feeling appears to be the general rule among many fasting patients. In nearly all cases, there is a much greater feeling of weakness in the advanced stages of prolonged fasting than at the beginning of the fast.

While recognizing the variation in strength and weakness during the fast, it should be understood that this is not an important determining factor in the recovery of most fasting patients. In any event strength which may have been lost on the fast is rapidly regained when food is again taken. Only in those very rare cases of extreme weakness need concern be given. Extreme emaciation, with weakness to the point of frequent fainting and inability to walk alone, is of course an indication that the fast should be broken.

A loss of weight while fasting is of course normal and to be expected. The average loss is perhaps about one pound a day, with a greater loss in the beginning of the fast than towards the end. Usually overweight patients lose weight most rapidly. Dr. Rabagliati and Dr. Carrington have reported cases in which a slight gain of weight was registered during short fasts. Such occurrences are very rare and difficult to explain.

There is of course no danger from the loss of weight while fasting; it is rapidly regained when eating is again resumed.

After the last meal is digested the digestive tract becomes inactive and there is usually very little bowel action. The intestines become empty, in fact, sterile, and bowel movements are infrequent or altogether absent. People have fasted as long as fifty days with no bowel action, and though this is exceptional, it indicates the tendency here given mention. The lack of frequent bowel action on the fast is quite normal and no cause for concern. Bowel action is quickly restored after the fast.

If and when bowel action does take place on the fast, the movements may be easy or difficult, depending in part on the type of food that was consumed immediately prior to the fast. Prof. Benedict stated that "fasting feces become hard, much drier and pillular, and frequently cause considerable uneasiness." This is true in some cases when the pre-fasting diet was composed predominately of refined and cooked foods. The use of an enema is then required to obtain relief. This condition does not tend to occur, however, when the meals immediately prior to the fast were composed exclusively of raw fruits and raw vegetables.

There is considerable variation in the sexual desire and activity of fasting patients. In most cases the desire is either reduced or abolished, with temporary impotency developing during long fasts. Occasionally patients continue to indulge sexually throughout the fast, and in rare cases fasting has produced an increase in the sexual desire. After the fast the sexual powers return with renewed vigor. Men who had been impotent prior to fasting have often regained virility, and sterility among women is also frequently corrected.

In women previously affected by congestion in the ovaries and uterus, the menses may appear at irregular intervals while fasting and appear almost viscid in consistency with an offensive odor. This is believed to result from the natural cleansing of the reproductive system. In most other cases the menses may be barely perceptible during the fast or it may not appear at all.

So long as good nutrition and habits of exercise are maintained after the fast, this same reduction or cessation in the menstrual discharge may be apparent. This need cause no concern or alarm, for the excessive flow from the uterus seen in civilized woman is the result of abnormal congestion in the reproductive system. When this congestion is relieved with fasting, the menstrual discharge is accordingly diminished.

To the most important symptoms given may be added literally dozens of others which may or may not occur, and which are quite unimportant insofar as the progress of the fast is concerned. Among these are vomiting, spitting crises, skin eruptions, headaches, backaches, dizziness, hiccoughs, fainting spells, sore throat, slight colds and cramps. Though such symptoms are discomforting to a degree, they are no cause for concern. Many are simply indicative of increased efforts of elimination. Of course, practically no patients experience all of these symptoms; many experience none at all, and others experience them on a few short periods during the fast.

The therapeutic action of the fast is exactly the opposite of that of drugs. Whereas the latter often suppress the symptoms of disease, it is the purpose of fasting to "bring out" such symptoms, eliminate all toxins present, and thus provide permanent recovery. A disease which in the past has been inactive, or suppressed with drugs, may become active through fasting, as tissues are healed and elimination increased. It has been said that we "have to live our diseases over again" while fasting, and this is true to the extent that the weakest parts of the body are being rejuvenated and cleansed, and thus given immediate renovative activity. People, for instance, who have been susceptible to catarrhal conditions in the past, may eliminate streams of mucus from the colon, vagina, throat, sinuses and nose, depending upon the location of their original catarrhal condition, while fasting. After elimination is complete, or the fast is broken, such symptoms cease and the patients are much the better for the experience, generally being cured of future catarrhal ailments. A disease may become more intense during the early days of fasting, and as renovation continues to completion, all symptoms gradually subside until the patient has fully recovered. Thus many, if not most, of the symptoms of fasting may be ascribed to the curative action of the fast itself. In no instance can we consider them the development of new pathology, as is shown by their rapid disappearance and failure to return after fasting.

Obviously this sort of analysis may give indication that the nature of disease itself is somewhat different than has been generally believed. In the past we have been accustomed to speak of disease as "attacking" the body as some sort of destructive force, and as such have attempted to "destroy" or suppress the disease itself with equally destructive agents, and even to remove the part of the body in which the disease was present. Here we see, in fasting, the action of disease as being curative in nature, which is intensified and brought to its culmination. Perhaps it is this which has induced many physicians who employed fasting to claim that disease itself may be a defensive mechanism that induces an "eliminative" crisis in the case of acute disease, or an "adaptive" crisis in the case of chronic disease. The validity of this concept remains to be seen, and it is not our purpose to consider it here, but rather to point out its relationship to the development of symptoms on the fast.

The most important danger signals of fasting, as regards the pulse and temperature, have been given, and there are but few other symptoms which may be considered sufficient reason for breaking the fast sooner than otherwise would be desired. Even temporary delirium on the fast (which has occurred seldom) is rarely considered as reason for giving food, unless the delirium is associated with heart palpitation. The palpitation of the heart itself, or pain in the heart, while fasting is quite uncommon and not considered dangerous. As a rule most symptoms of the fast must be considered in relation to others. Very few symptoms in themselves are sufficient reason for breaking the fast. It is the combination of many severe symptoms which, even though not always dangerous, is occasionally used as a reason for giving food. There are no hard and fast rules in this respect, and each physician must use his own judgment in considering a particular case.

The symptoms of fasting, quite apart from being a cause for worry or concern, can thus be seen to be only outward manifestations of the gradual recovery to health being made. Few are seriously discomforting, and one symptom, the loss of hunger, even makes the fast much more pleasant. In the final analysis, it is hunger itself which is most dreaded on the fast, and when this disappears, fasting is quite easy, with little annoyance or discomfort. Certainly it is not so difficult an ordeal as going through continued ill health, and many do not look upon it as an "ordeal" at all, but rather enjoy their fast to an extent not commonly expected.

❧ VIII ☙

Supervising the Fast

GREAT CARE is taken in the administration of most therapeutic agents. Many forms of medication can be very
dangerous if used by the layman without complete knowledge of technique and quantity. Massage, manipulation and
other forms of physical therapy can be useless when not properly applied. Fasting is no exception to this principle in the
sense that certain precautions must be taken by all patients.
These are not as complex as one often finds in the field of
medicine, and ignoring them usually does not have the disastrous consequences found in the misuse of other therapeutic
agents. Yet both physician and layman should recognize certain fundamental rules which permit supervision of fasting
at maximum efficiency and a minimum degree of danger.

No form of preparatory treatment is essential to the fast,
though one type of dietary change is helpful and will render
the fast more effective. The highly refined and heat-processed
foods of the conventional diet have a tendency to clog the intestinal tract. If the fast begins at a time when excessive
amounts of food residue are packed against the walls of the
small intestine and colon, the patient may experience some gas
and difficulty of bowel exacuation, and the efficiency of the fast
may be lowered. This tends to be prevented if the patient consumes an abundance of raw food, especially in the form of
juicy fruits and succulent vegetables, immediately prior to the
fast. As a rule, living upon raw fruits and vegetables for just a
day or two before the fast will loosen the bowels considerably

and promote copious elimination when this is necessary. With the alimentary canal thus cleaner and free from excessive residues, the fast will be more comfortable and effective. The raw fruit-vegetable diet also serves the purpose of accustoming the system to the reduced intake of concentrated foods, thus making possible the easiest transition into the absolute fast. In the case of certain acute diseases, in which there is no appetite and normal digestion is impossible, the fast should begin at once and preparatory dietary measures would not be in order. But for a planned fast in non-emergency cases, the brief dietary preparation as indicated will be found helpful.

Rest is the first recommendation to all fasting patients. Some physicians require rest in bed in all cases of fasting, and whereas this is perhaps taking the extreme attitude, it is founded upon a sound physiological basis. Observations made during many long fasts show that the active individual consumes his nutritive reserves and energy more rapidly than the patient who rests most of the time. The resting patient can fast longer and emerges from the fast in better condition.

People have often worked throughout long fasts. In one instance a New York athlete received considerable attention by walking cross-country over 500 miles during 20 days of fasting. No permanent harm was observed in this or similar cases and satisfactory results were obtained. The question here is not what is necessary, but what is advisable. Both active and resting individuals receive benefit from fasting, though the latter perhaps recover more rapidly and are more comfortable during the fast.

During short fasts, less than 10 days in duration, doing light work, and perhaps even taking a few exercises, should be quite harmless. Even on longer fasts some very light work or exercise may be permitted, but caution is much more important in such cases. The important thing here is to avoid excesses. The patient who is weak at the start of the fast can obviously be less active than the athlete or strong individual. Providing activity is not carried to the point of excessive weakness or exhaustion, the efficiency of the fast is perhaps not impaired. However, Puriton's recommendations of "loafing, resting, lazing along and not caring" are perhaps most appealing to any fasting patient, from the standpoint of comfort alone, and whenever possible the fast should be conducted accordingly.

The second important need of fasting patients is warmth. This is especially true in the advanced stages of fasting, when the patient can freeze to death at temperatures which normally would be found only a little discomforting. Also, lack of warmth probably impedes the process of elimination to a degree and interferes with the efficiency of the fast.

If the patient continually complains of being too hot, but has cold extremities, the fast should be broken and artificial heat applied. In event of an extreme chill the fast should not be continued and all efforts must be made to provide sufficient warmth. Under normal conditions, with proper care, conditions such as these do not arise, but when, through carelessness, warmth is not maintained, especially during prolonged fasts, the precautions given mention should have immediate and careful attention.

Many fasting institutions employ sunbathing with fasting. The beneficial effects of exposure to sunlight have long been well-known and sunbathing is no doubt helpful to the patient. However, it is very important to avoid extremes in this respect. Sunbaths should always be of comparatively short duration during the fast. A sunstroke is possible when there is excessive exposure, and whereas there is generally rapid recovery in such cases, a little care is certain to prevent them in the first place. While fasting it is always best to take the sunbaths during the early morning and late afternoon when the temperature is not at its highest. As the fast progresses, the length of the sunbaths should gradually be decreased.

It is particularly important to avoid fear and negative mental influences while fasting. The ill effects of anger, grief and shock are more pronounced while fasting than at any other time. Sinclair remarks that the faster "should not have about him terrified aunts and cousins who will tell him that he looks like a corpse, that his pulse is below forty and that his heart may stop beating in the night." Certainly this is true in all cases, and a group of well-meaning friends and relatives can be a great interference to the efficiency of fasting when they have no knowledge or understanding of the purposes and principles of the fast. If for reason of the environment, or other reasons, the patient is living in dread and fear of the consequences of fasting, the fast should not be continued.

Cleanliness and fresh air are important during the fast just as at all other times. During bathing, extremes of temperature should be avoided, and the bath should not last too long. When the patient is very weak, a sponge bath only should be used. There should be fresh air in the room whenever possible, though in cold climates this should not be carried to the point of interfering with warmth.

There has been some controversy as to the amount of water to drink while fasting. Theoretical observers have advocated water-free fasts, and still others have recommended several quarts of water a day on the fast. Experienced physicians have not gone to such extremes, but have instead recommended thirst as a reliable guide. There is little doubt but what several quarts of water a day while fasting is greatly in excess of actual needs, and hence probably impedes elimination. Water-free fasts, on the other hand, are dangerous and should never be employed. There are no records of anyone living longer than seventeen days with neither food nor water. A certain amount of water may be regarded as essential on every long fast. Fasting two or three days without water probably does no harm, but longer fasts in the absence of water are inadvisable. The actual desire for water on a fast is usually not great, but can be relied upon to meet all needs. It usually calls for about a pint to a quart or two of water each day, depending upon each individual case. Occasionally days may arise on the fast in which no water is desired, in which case none need be taken if the length of time does not exceed a few days. It may be added that spring water or tested well water is to be recommended while fasting. Distilled water may be a second choice, whereas chlorinated water should be avoided if any other form is available.

A certain amount of debate has also centered about the use of the enema while fasting. Though the enema has been widely used in some fasting institutions, most experienced physicians today either refrain from using it altogether or use it very seldom. Recommendations of the enema are based upon the assumption that toxins and waste matter are being deposited in the colon during the fast, and that the same materials are in turn re-absorbed by the blood. Cleansing the lower bowel with an enema each day supposedly prevents such re-absorption.

Actually the colon is not fundamentally an organ from which much absorption occurs, and experienced physicians have noted that the entire alimentary canal, including the colon, becomes quite free of all waste materials during the fast. There is no evidence to indicate that the supposed deposits in the colon occur. The use of the enema is to some degree a drain on the patient's vitality, which is already at a low ebb. It also washes away the mucus which normally protects the lining of the colon, and it breaks some of the tiny muscles of the intestinal wall, thus causing the muscle tone to be damaged and laying the groundwork for future constipation. It has further been noticed that bowel action is usually restored more rapidly after the fast when the enema has not been used.

In spite of these criticisms, there are occasionally circumstances which do indicate the limited use of the enema while fasting. If the diet immediately prior to the fast was largely cooked and refined, and the feces become hard and dried out on the fast, an enema can be used to remove the fecal matter. This helps to prevent the formation of gas and will eliminate difficulty and pain during bowel evacuation. In the case of hemorrhoid patients, it will prevent a hard plug of feces from forming in the rectal tissues. It must be pointed out, however, that even with poor diet prior to fasting, hard fecal matter, with difficulty in passing, does not always occur. Further, if the meals immediately prior to the fast were composed exclusively of raw fruits and raw vegetables, as has been previously recommended, this adverse condition may be prevented in nearly all cases, including those of hemorrhoid patients. If solid foods, in particular those which have been heat-processed, are taken too soon after fasting, bowel action may also be rendered difficult and use of an enema may be called for. Here again we find an easily preventable condition, which does not tend to occur if the fast is broken in the right manner. It is thus apparent that the enema is very rarely necessary during or after a properly conducted fast. Its use is indicated in exceptional cases only, and then it should be applied just often enough to provide relief for such adverse symptoms as may be present.

It is important to avoid all forms of drugs while fasting, as these are readily absorbed by the patient, who in turn does not handle them as well as the normal individual. The danger of drugs on the fast was noted in particular by Aducco, when fasting dogs were given cocaine, strychnine and phenol. In all cases the reactions were much more intense than when doses were given to well-nourished animals, with a rapid rise in temperature, pronounced motor reflexes, and occasionally violent convulsions resulting in such cases. Delafuoy also found that fasting animals are very sensitive to drugs, and Mansfield reported that drugs which produced only slight effects on ordinary rabbits, produced severe reactions and violent convulsions when given to the animals while fasting. Other investigators indicate similar results, and with humans an equal sensitivity to drugs while fasting must be expected.

Serums and injections of all forms must also be avoided while fasting, as is the case with different methods of physical therapy, such as spinal manipulations, gastric lavages, Turkish baths, cold baths, electrical treatments, etc. The fasting cure does not harmonize well with a variety of other therapeutic measures. Most of these are a further drain on the patient's vitality, and in the cases of serum or vaccine injections, there is extreme danger with possible death. It must be remembered that the physiological effects of fasting are the exact opposite in many respects of those of other therapeutic agents. A combination of such methods, quite apart from being useless, only produces complex reactions which tend to contradict each other.

It can be seen that therapeutic fasting is complete in itself. It is not a procedure which is to be used along with too many adjuncts and other therapeutic devices. The principles of its technique are few and render its application both safe and practical. With a reasonable degree of care, the fasting patient may pass through a comfortable period of therapeutic treatment and regain health in the most effective and pleasant manner.

✒ IX ✒

Breaking the Fast

O<small>F</small> <small>VITAL IMPORTANCE</small> to the fasting patient is the
method of breaking the fast. The period of abstinence
may be completely successful, but if this is not terminated
properly the results can be decidedly unfavorable. Many lay-
men have conducted their fasts with the greatest care, only to
break them on whatever food happened to be most convenient
and find themselves in dire distress. A few physicians, unfa-
miliar with the general technique of fasting, have likewise
broken fasts in an experimental or careless manner, and found
their patients to react in the most alarming fashion. To give
inadequate attention to this matter is to court near-disaster;
it may mean the difference in certain cases between life and
death.

The many reports of fasts which have been broken incor-
rectly well substantiate this and give vivid illustration of the
possible aftermaths. Dr. Shelton refers to two fasts broken by
an incompetent physician on chocolate candy, which were
followed by extreme gastric and intestinal acidity and great
distress throughout the body. He refers to another fast broken
on toast, followed by malnutritional edema. Dr. Havard
recorded a case in which a 28 day fast was broken on a meal
of beefsteak, potatoes, bread and butter, after which violent
vomiting spells occurred, with inability to retain even water
which was afterwards given. He writes of another fast, 42
days in duration, broken on coarse bread, and followed by
vomiting and extreme irritation of the stomach. Another

report tells of a 31 day fast, broken on several beef sandwiches, followed by death.

Prof. Ehret has pointed to a fast by a diabetic patient, broken on dates, which ended fatally. A different case described by Ehret involved a 28 day fast, broken on boiled potatoes. An operation was necessary to remove the food, which was held in the contracted intestines, after which the patient died. Sinclair writes of a man "who fasted fifty days, and then ate half a dozen figs, and caused intestinal abrasions from which he lost a great deal of blood." Regarding one of his own fasts, Sinclair states that it was broken on a thoroughly ripe Japanese persimmon which "doubled me up with the most alarming cramp—and in consequence I do not recommend persimmons for fasters."

When intake of food is stopped, the body adjusts itself to the new conditions. The digestive organs cease to exercise their natural function; the digestive glands do not produce the usual juices, and the stomach itself shrinks to much less than its usual size. All this is an associated requirement of the physiological rest.

After many days of fasting the body thus loses its immediate power to digest and handle food in the usual manner. When foods are again taken it only gradually regains its power of normal function. If the first intake is of a solid nature and difficult of digestion, the organs may entirely rebel; there will be little or no digestive activity, and the foods will decay and ferment, causing much distress and discomfort. If this happens along the lower section of the digestive tract, in the small intestine, the reactions are most severe, and when peristaltic action to move the food is yet impossible, death may ensue.

Hence the reason for selecting foods with the utmost care after the fast. With few exceptions there is general unanimity of opinion that the first nutriment should be of a liquid nature, for it thus is more rapidly absorbed and is easier of digestion. It is also more soothing and less abrasive to the delicate mucous membrane lining, which is especially sensitive at this time.

Fruit and vegetables juices, vegetable broths, flesh broths and milk have all been employed. They have not, however, given equally satisfactory results. Milk is too difficult of digestion for some patients immediately after the fast, and, if taken in large amounts, it is not always assimilated without trouble and tends to delay the return of normal bowel action. Flesh broths have other disadvantages, and after long fasts they may give adverse reactions, even though there is ease of digestion. The strained broth of cooked vegetables is much better, but of widest use and generally most satisfactory results are the uncooked juices of fresh fruits and vegetables. Discomfort is practically unknown when these foods are used. There is ease of digestion, rapid assimiliation and quick restoration of bowel elimination.

Though both are practical, fruit juices are usually chosen over those of vegetables for breaking the fast. Unstrained orange juice is given preference by most practitioners, especially for the first few feedings, and it provides perhaps the easiest and most effective return of normal bowel action. Juices of the grapefruit, tomato, grape, pineapple, peach, pear, apricot, apple, cantaloupe, watermelon, strawberry and other juicy fruits may also be used, either to break the fast or to supplement orange juice after the fast is broken. Of vegetable products, carrot juice is considered most appropriate at this time.

The fast should be broken on one-half glass of juice, followed by the same amount every hour, or by one glass every two hours, for the rest of the day. On the second day the same schedule may be followed, or the juices may be taken at less frequent intervals; a three-meal-a-day plan may be adopted if desired, about one pint of juice being taken at each meal. On the following days the quantity of juice taken may be increased, but care must always be taken to avoid excesses which might produce digestive discomfort. At no time on the post-fasting juice diet should more than an approximate pint of juice be taken at any one feeding.

The best uncooked juices for use after the fast are freshly extracted. This is true for reason of palatability as well as nutrition. The sweetness and richness of flavor of freshly extracted
juices are especially acceptable for the post-fasting patient.
Within minutes after being made, however, juices tend to lose
their fine flavors through the process of oxidation. Enzymes,
vitamins and other nutrients are lost in the same way. For this
reason, all forms of bottled juices, which were prepared long
before consumption, should be avoided after fasting provided
some form of fresh juice is available.

The juices used immediately after the fast are best served at
room temperature, which permits easiest digestion. Cold and
iced juices should always be avoided at this time. The first juices
should be sipped very slowly. If they are consumed in great
haste, without proper insalivation, stomach cramps and the
formation of gas can result. If the juices are "chewed" before
being swallowed, the acid and sugar of the fruit will be mixed
with saliva and work of the stomach will be reduced to a minimum.

The duration of the juice diet may vary from one to approximately six days, depending primarily upon the length of the
fast. Whereas the juice diet increases in length in accordance
with the extension of the fast, the rate of increase is a decreasing
one. The ratio of the fast to the juice diet may be only two or
three to one in the case of very short fasts, about four or five to
one in the case of fasts of moderate duration, and seven to one
or greater in the case of very long fasts. This is expressed in full
in the following chart, which represents a suggested time schedule for correlating the juice diet with the length of the fast.

Length of Fast	Length of Juice Diet
1 to 3 days	1 day
4 to 8 days	2 days
9 to 15 days	3 days
16 to 24 days	4 days
25 to 35 days	5 days
over 35 days	6 days

This chart represents a general guide and not a specific rule. Certain deviations may be made under different circumstances. The patient who shows a long history of digestive weakness, constipation or hemorrhoids can occasionally profit from a slightly longer juice diet than usual. On the other hand, some people need not employ the juice diet quite as long as others who have fasted an equal length of time, and after "complete" fasts of long duration, there is customarily a reduction in duration of the juice diet. If hunger returns while fasting, salivary secretion is normalized and other digestive secretions are becoming available at the very time the fast is broken. Solid foods can then be handled somewhat sooner than when incomplete fasts of the same duration are broken. The earlier introduction of solid nutriment in these cases is also helpful because the food reserves of the body are in need of more rapid replacement. In view of these considerations, the time factor of each juice regime should be treated in relation to all of the individual physical factors present, as well as the length and physiological stage of the fast.

Following the juice diet all types of uncooked foods may be eaten. A slow transition to a normal diet is unnecessary if the juices are consumed for the recommended length of time and if the normal diet thereafter is composed exclusively of uncooked foods. If, however, a variety of heat-processed foodstuffs are to be consumed, the uncooked dietary should be adopted first and may serve as a transition diet. This should be continued at least as long as the juice diet itself. It may also be continued permanently to assure optimum benefit from the fast when this course of dietary procedure is decided upon.

The first regular meals following the juice diet should be small in size. On successive days the quantity of food may be gradually increased. However, care must be taken to avoid excesses. A gradual transition into very large meals, to compensate for previous restrictions, is definitely not called for. Moderation in eating is always desirable, and this is more important following a period of prolonged abstinence than at other times. Equally important is the proper mastication of all foodstuffs.

Liquids should be sipped slowly and solid foods should be chewed to the point of involuntary swallowing. Adequate attention to these factors will prevent overtaxing the digestive organs at a time when they are regaining their full working capacity.

The importance of breaking the fast properly can hardly be overestimated. Certainly more difficulties have resulted from incorrect breaking of the fast than from any other form of fasting mismanagement. Yet these difficulties can easily be avoided in all cases. We need only remember that the proper application of the uncooked juice diet is the basic key to success in the immediate post-fasting period. When this is followed by a varied dietary of uncooked foods, consumed in moderate quantities and well masticated, the normal physiological adjustment of the body is completed in an ideal manner.

❧ X ❧

Living after the Fast

THE PURPOSE of therapeutic fasting is to remove the causes of ill health. Once these causes are removed, the various manifestations of disease which were present tend to disappear and the patient is said to have recovered. However, just as faulty living habits created the causes of illness in the first place, so can these same living habits, if continued after fasting, create the conditions which may produce disease all over again.

There is no therapeutic agent of any nature which is certain to offer a permanent remedy of disease if no thought is given to the mode of living after the agent is used. Most therapeutic methods, in fact, fail to preserve health permanently irrespective of the mode of living which follows their use. The suppression of symptoms with drugs, for instance, or the use of vaccine and serum therapy, are not even expected by those who employ them to remove the causes of disease. They are expected to exert important influences which will aid the patient, it is true, but in few instances can their results be expected to be permanent.

Thus fasting, though its results are more permanent than is the usual rule in therapeutics, does not make one "disease-proof" in the sense that the conditions which favor the development of disease cannot be built all over again. There are manifestations of disease that disappear during the fast and never return, no matter how the patient lives thereafter. There

69

are other diseases that return rapidly after a fast if the mode of living is not correct. The determining factors in such cases are many and involve the character and type of disease present, and its stage of development, as well as the strength and general vitality of the patient. On the other hand, if care is taken to adhere to good living habits, a true control is made over the preservation of good health; permanence of recovery from specific manifestations of disease may be regarded as probable, and in many cases, virtually certain.

There are many theories as to the causes of ill health. These may be grouped into four main categories—chemical, bacterial, mechanical and mental. Whereas it is not to be denied that each of these is of some importance in determining the state of physical well-being, the preponderance of scientific knowledge seems to favor the viewpoint that it is primarily chemistry which dominates the efficiency of physiological functions in the body, with bacterial, mechanical and mental conditions acting chiefly as secondary causes, being dependent upon the initial chemical condition of the body. It is not our object here to go into detail regarding this matter, but simply to state that this assumption as to the causes of disease is generally accepted by physicians who employ fasting and that their consideration of the care of patients after fasting is determined accordingly.

Basically the chemistry of the body is determined by nutrition. Sunshine, exercise, fresh air, mental tranquility, as well as other factors, are also of some importance. The initial intake of minerals, vitamins and other vital elements is made through our consumption of food. Sunshine adds vitamin D and also seems to act as a catalytic agent which creates certain changes in the chemistry of the blood, with the calcium and phosphorus content in particular increased during sunbaths. It thus appears that sunshine may induce the secretion of certain hormones or ferments which permit the body to use certain chemicals that it otherwise would not be able to use. Exercise stimulates the functional activities throughout the body, increases the supply of oxygen through deep breathing, and increases the flow of nutritive matter to the cells. The purity of air is important, with many harmful toxins being taken into the lungs when the atmosphere of cities is infiltrated with smoke and smog from industrial plants. Emotional reactions may alter the activity of various glands and stimulate or decrease their internal secretions, as the case may be.

Defective nutrition after the fast results in part from consuming foods that have been altered chemically during the processes of refining, cooking, canning and pasteurization. Refined foods have lost the greater part of their mineral and vitamin content, and marked amounts of these elements are lost when foods are heated. Even prolonged storage often causes important losses of elements in foods. Many kinds of chemical treatment are also destructive, with the bleaching of flour, vegetables and other foods, insecticide spraying of many plants, sulphuring of dried fruits, and chemical additions to many meats and canned foods having the most marked effects. Many chemicals, in addition to or instead of lowering the food value, give toxic reactions in the body as well, especially when taken in large amounts.

In the case of cooking there occur a number of chemical changes which are probably just as important as the losses of minerals and vitamins. Tars are formed in all foods which are scorched by heat until black forms on the outside. Such tars have been found to be carcinogenic when tested under experimental conditions, and hence they represent a serious objection to certain heat-processed foods. It is well known that all enzymes are heat-labile. Even the comparatively low heating temperature used in pasteurizing milk destroys every enzyme in the food. Certain hormones are also affected by heat, as are the essential amino acids comprising the protein of foods. Some of the amino acids, such as lysine and glutamine, are destroyed; others are denatured and become less valuable for nutritive purposes. The total protein fraction is coagulated by heat and rendered less digestible. Fats may be damaged even more, and

much experimental evidence is available showing that they
may become carcinogenic after prolonged treatment at high
temperatures. Probably all of the activating substances and
vitalizing factors of food are changed to some extent under sufficient exposure to heat. The complex chemical balance of all
food nutrients is altered, with the entire physico-chemical
change being sufficient to produce serious physical impairment
among those consuming large amounts of the foods.

This is clearly shown, under different conditions, by both
animal experiment and human experience. Under carefully
controlled conditions, natural foods of almost every description
have been tested and re-tested for their effects upon the health
of white rats, guinea pigs, cats, dogs, monkeys and other experimental animals. And the results have consistently shown that
raw fruits, raw vegetables, raw nuts and other seed foods, raw
honey, raw dairy products and raw meat products (selected according to animal types) all produce much better results upon
animal health than do their counterparts in heat-processed
form. Animals fed exclusively upon uncooked foods mantain a
state of splendid health, with practically no signs of physical,
mental, sexual or reproductive impairment. Animals of the
same species fed a similar selection of foods, only in heat-processed form, develop literally dozens of pathological symptoms.
These include severe degenerative diseases, as well as physical
deformities in the new-born, behavior disturbances, sexual ab-
normalities, reproductive impairment and shortened life spans.
The most common bacterial and virus diseases, together with
parasitic infestations, are very common in cooked-fed animals
and almost unknown in animals fed selected uncooked foods.
The mortality rate is always much higher when heat-processed
foods are provided. Eventually, if sufficient cooked foods are included in the diet of certain animals over many generations,
reproduction itself becomes impossible and the strains of animal
stock completely die out.

With humans the effects are less severe in terms of survival,
but they are quite similar in terms of certain manifestations of

bodily impairment. In some instances the rate of diseases in white rats fed selected heat-processed foods has been found to correspond almost exactly with the average incidence of the same diseases in human groups using approximately the same foods. In the civilized world the widespread use of refined, heat-processed and otherwise damaging foodstuffs has its effects in the extremely high incidence of degenerative diseases and mental disturbances. Despite the widespread availability of medical services, and nationwide efforts towards control of our common diseases, most signs of physical and mental deterioration are increasing in number, in some instances at a rapid rate. Certain infectious conditions are also becoming more common, and we are now faced with the wide prevalency of new virus and fungus diseases which previously were almost unknown. Parturition has become so painful and complicated that it is described in terms of a pathological process. Birth defects rise in incidence with each succeeding generation, as does mental retardation in young children. In adult life there is frequent incomplete development of secondary sexual characteristics, and other imperfections of physique are usually so common as to be taken for granted.

What a remarkable contrast we then find among different primitive racial groups which retained their native dietary habits into a recent era, using no refined foods and a smaller percentage of those which had been cooked. Scientists observed and studied isolated and semi-isolated groups of such people and found them to be enjoying a state of health unheard of in civilization. Under the most adequate nutritional conditions of primitive life, dental decay was entirely absent; the dental arches were of perfect form and regularity; infectious diseases were quite rare, and some of the degenerative processes were entirely unknown. Parturition was painless, or nearly so, with scarcely any complications. Birth defects were extremely rare, and the secondary sexual characteristics of men and women were fully developed. At the same time chemical analysis of the foods utilized in primitive life showed a content of minerals and vitamins many times as high as is normally found in modern foods. Some of the typical primitive diets of the healthiest tribal groups were found to contain over ten times the amount of fat-soluble vitamins as in the displacing diets, with the proportion of certain minerals being from five to twenty-five times as high.

This all finds a very important correlation with the experiences of patients after a period of fasting. Those who once again return to the conventional diet—this largely refined and heat-processed—often receive the surprise and disappointment of seeing their old diseases, which disappeared on the fast, return in the same intensity and manner. In the nineteenth century era of fasting, when the science of nutrition was in its early experimental stages, physicians often gave little thought to the patient's diet after fasting, and the problem of obtaining a permanent cure was then very real. Today the relation between fasting and nurtition is well recognized, and the usual patient is given careful instructions for eating after the fast.

The general nutritional requirement may be stated as follows. To the degree that foods are grown on fertile, biologically-active soil (developed and maintained primarily by adequate mulching practices), without the use of caustic chemical fertilizers or poisonous pesticides, are they suitable in terms of flavor, nutritive qualities and safety for use in the human food supply. And to the degree that foods of all basic types are used in their relatively natural state, without chemical adulteration, refining or heat-processing, are they adapted to support life and maintain immunity to disease. It is the purpose of fasting to restore health; it is then the purpose of scientific nutrition, with other hygienic factors, to maintain it. After the fast, the diet should be both unrefined and uncooked to as great an extent as possible. In view of the present chemical and radioactive contamination of our physical environment, including our food supply, this step is not certain to provide the perfect nutrition that was once attainable, but it will give the best nutrition possible within the framework that exists. While not ideal, this is still sufficient for the purposes in question. For some patients after fasting, an adequate food stock may be available and an excellent nutritional basis may be established. Others will doubtless deviate from the optimum nutritional standard, but all can keep the general goals of scientific nutrition in mind and endeavor to follow them as much as possible.

Though correct diet is important as a permanent phase of living after the fast, it is especially so for the first few weeks or months, when the body is regaining normal weight. During this period a very high percentage of nutriment is being absorbed from the food, and if the new protoplasm being built is to be healthy and biologically adequate, the source material must be of high quality. If reconstruction is made entirely from the same foods which rendered the body ill in the first place, the eventual advantages of the fast may be virtually nullified. Once the body weight is stabilized, and maintenance is the only requirement, the food will cease to be so vital a determining factor, though it will still affect the health in a very definite manner and should be selected with care.

Many are disappointed to learn that permanence of recovery resulting from fasting is very largely dependent upon their manner of living thereafter, with particular emphasis upon dietary habits. The fast is regarded as a sufficiently trying ordeal in itself, without having to undertake special restrictions or health measures thereafter. Upon conclusion of the fast, however, such disappointment is almost entirely absent. The appetite is sharpened, and pleasure is obtained from consuming foods which may formerly have been avoided. The total uncooked diet not only becomes a delight to the sense of taste, but usually affords more satisfaction than a conventional mode of eating did prior to the fast.

These new-found culinary pleasures are of course dependent upon sufficient variety in the uncooked diet, as well as interesting methods of preparing the foods in use. And they can be dependent to some degree upon the sources of food products. Although poor quality foods derived from chemically treated soil or artificial animal feeding practices will provide more flavor in an uncooked diet than they would in a conventional diet, they still tend to be rather dull and flat tasting in comparison to foods produced under ideal conditions. It has frequently been noted, for instance, that fruits, berries, vegetables and nuts produced with suitable mulching methods of soil care have indescribably more delicacy, richness and perfection of flavor than do ordinary plant products. For this reason, an uncooked diet in which properly produced foods are found is a source of particular pleasure during the post-fasting period, although it is not necessarily indispensible to an acceptable level of culinary satisfaction.

So long as correct nutrition is maintained after the fast do the proper foods remain enjoyable and satisfying. There is generally no desire or craving for highly refined foodstuffs, and even the want for alcoholic beverages and tobacco may have disappeared. If change is then made, however, back to a more conventional mode of nutrition, this ceases to hold true and many of the old desires return. Appetite is chiefly a result of habit, and though it can be normalized by fasting, it can again be restored to a condition of abnormality and perversion, insofar as the associated intake of food supplies, in adequate measure, the nutritional needs of the body.

Fasting thus must be recognized only as a means of promoting the remedy of disease and the creation of health. It is not a method of maintaining health. This depends, as it always has, with both man and animals, upon the general hygienic factors of proper nutrition, sunlight, exercise, pure air, etc. The purpose of fasting is basically therapeutic, and in this sense it not only meets the requirements of most patients, but is perhaps the most effective measure ever to be employed.

Clearly the extraordinary value of fasting has not been recognized by the professions of healing as a whole. In spite of the careful scientific work done with fasting by physiologists, biologists and physicians, and the almost universal recommendation of the method by these people, orthodox medicine has scarcely recognized that fasting even has therapeutic properties or has been used for any other purpose than a religious rite. The ordinary physician is as completely unaware of fasting as is the layman. Hence the purpose of this short treatise. Here we have covered some of the important points of fasting, which may serve to incite inquiry for further investigation among physician and layman alike, and perhaps to some degree act as a limited guide in the employment of fasting for therapeutic purposes.

Bibliography

1. ALLEN, F. N., *Control of experimental diabetes by fasting and total dietary restriction.* J. Exp. Med., 31, 575-86, 1920
2. ALSAKER, R., *The master key to health.* East Aurora, N. Y., Sun-Diet Health Foundation, 1933
3. ASH, J. E., *The blood in inanition.* Arch. inter. Med., 14: 8-32, July, 1914
4. BASSLER, A., *The fasting cure answered.* Month. Cycle & Med. Bull. 4:332-334
5. BEAN, C. H., *Starvation and mental development.* Psychol. Clin., 3, 78-85, 1908
6. BENEDICT, F. G., *The influence of inanition on metabolism.* Publications, Carnegie Institution, Washington, 1907
7. BENEDICT, F. G., *A Study of prolonged fasting.* Publications, Carnegie Institution, Washington, 1915
8. CARLSON, A. J., *The control of hunger in health and disease.* Chicago, 1916
9. CARLSON, A. J., *Hunger, appetite and gastric juice secretion in man during prolonged fasting.* Am. J. Physiol., 45, 120-46, 1918
10. CARRINGTON, H., *Vitality, fasting, and nutrition.* New York, Rebman Co., 1908
11. CARRINGTON, H., *Fasting for health and long life.* Mokelumne Hill, Calif., Health Research, 1953
12. McCOY, F., *The fast way to health.* Los Angeles, McCoy Publications, 1938
13. CHILD, C. M., *Senescence and rejuvenescence.* The University of Chicago Press, 1915
14. CLEMMESEN, C., *Inanition and epilepsy: studies on the influence of inanition upon epileptic attacks.* Copenhagen, Levin and Munksgaard, 1932
15. DEWEY, E. H., *The true science of living.* London, Henry Bill Pub. Co., 1895
16. DEWEY, E. H., *The no-breakfast plan and the fasting cure.* London, L. N. Fowler & Co., 1900

17. EHRET, A., *Rational fasting*. Los Angeles, Ehret Pub. Co., 1926

18. FRAZIER, B. C., *Prolonged starvation*. Louisville, Month. J. Med. and Surg., 15:147-254, 1908

19. GORDON, *A prolonged fast*. Montreal Med. J., 36-482, 1907

20. GRAHAM, S., *The science of human life*. New York, Fowler and Wells, 1843

21. GUELPA, A., *Starvation and purgation in the relief of disease*. Brit. Med. J., 2:1050, 1910

22. GUELPA, A., *Autointoxication and disintoxication*. New York, Rebman Co.

23. HAY, W. H., *Health via food*. East Aurora, N. Y., Sun-Diet Health Foundation, 1929

24. HAY, W. H., *A new health era*. Mount Pocano, Pa., 1933

25. HAZZARD, L. B., *Fasting for the cure of disease*. Physical Culture Pub. Co., 1910

26. HAZZARD, L. B., *Scientific fasting*. New York, Grant Pub., 1927

27. HOWE, P. E., and HAWK, P. B., *Nitrogen partition and physiological resistance as influenced by repeated fasting*. J. Am. Chemical Soc., 33:215-254, 1910

28. HOWE, P. E., and HAWK, P. B., *A metabolism study on a fasting man*. Proc. Am. Soc. Biol. Chem., 31, 1912

29. HOWE, P. E., and HAWK, P. B., *On the differential leucocyte count during prolonged fasting*. Am. J. Physiol., 30: 174-181, 1912

30. LANGFIELD, H. S., *On the psychophysiology of a prolonged fast*. Psychol. Monogr., 16:5, 1914

31. MACFADDEN, B. A., *Fasting for health*. Macfadden Publications, 1923

32. McEACHEN, J., *Fasting for better health*. Escondido, Calif., J. McEachen, 1957

33. MELTZER, S., and MORRIS, C. H., *On the influence of*

fasting upon the bacteriological action of the blood. J. Exp. Med., 4:131-135, 1889

34. MEYERS, A. W., *Some morphological effects of prolonged inanition.* J. Med. Research, 36:51-77, 1917

35. MINOT, C. S., *Senescence and rejuvenation.* J. Physiol., 12:97-153, 1891

36. MORGULIS, S., *Contributions to the physiology of regeneration.* J. Exp. Zool., 7:595-642, 1909

37. MORGULIS, S., *Fasting and undernutrition.* E. P. Dutton & Co., 1923

38. OLDFIELD, J., *Fasting for health and life.* London, C. W. Daniel Co., 1924

39. PATON, N. D., and STOCKMAN, R., *Observations on the metabolism of a fasting man.* Royal Soc. Edinburgh, 4:3, 1889

40. PENNY, F., *Notes on a thirty day fast.* Brit. Med. J., 1: 1414-16, 1909

41. PURINTON, E. E., *Philosophy of fasting.* New York, Lust Pub., 1906

42. SANDS, N. J., *Prolonged fasting as a factor in the treatment of acute disease, with special reference to affections of the alimentary canal.* N. Y. State J. Med., 4:55, 1904

43. SHELTON, H. M., *The hygienic system,* vol. 3, Dr. Shelton's Health School, San Antonio, 1934

44. SHELTON, H. M., *The hygienic system,* vol. 7, Dr. Shelton's Health School, San Antonio, 1941

45. SINCLAIR, U. P., *The fasting cure.* M. Kennerly, 1913

46. STERN, H., *Fasting and undernutrition in the treatment of diabetes.* New York, Rebman Co., 1912

47. SWEET, M. P., *Hints on fasting well.* Mokelumne Hill, Calif., Health Research, 1956

48. SZEKELY, E. B., *The therapeutics of fasting.* Tecate, 1942

49. TILDEN, J. M., *Criticisms of the practice of medicine,* 1909

50. WEGER, G. S., *The genesis and control of disease.* Los Angeles, 1931

INDEX

81

-ADDENDUM-

This material contains much valuable information. The Shangri-La Health Resort, however, does not necessarily endorse every statement in it. Contentious matters should be submitted in the form of a question with sufficient money to cover the cost of a reply.

This material is distributed by The Shangri-La Health Resort as a part of their educational program. Speakers on natural health are also available for group meetings. (Transportation and lodging must be provided.) A complete current catalogue of "The Shangri-La selection" of books, tapes and pamphlets on natural health and better living will be sent on request and the payment of twenty-five cents in stamps or coin.

The Shangri-La offers a learn-by-doing educational program in normal living and total well-being for all who are interested in a better way of life. Weight reducing, fasting, exercise programs, and choice natural organic foods (when available) will enable you to build better health. We have our own organic gardens and fruit grove.

Regular lectures, personal consultations, and discussions with other natural living student guests will help you to acquire a better understanding of how to prevent disease. A library, sunbathing solariums, boating from our own private docks, regular trips to nearby beaches, heated swimming pool, and other recreational facilities are all available for your enjoyment at no additional charge.

The sunny climate, lovely grounds, and choice facilities at The Shangri-La make learning and relaxing an easy pleasure. The cost is moderate. Cooperative working arrangements are available for those who wish to work for part or all of their expenses.

Write for free picture brochure and complete information.

THE SHANGRI-LA HEALTH RESORT
Bonita Springs, Florida 33923